# APPENDIX
(1925)

# APPENDIX
## (1925)

POLAK
NOVAK
SCHUMANN
NEWELL
NORRIS
FRANK
EHRENFEST
LYNCH
KOSMAK
CHILD
GELLHORN
DAVIS
TAUSSIG
CULBERTSON
RUBIN

# GYNECOLOGICAL AND OBSTETRICAL MONOGRAPHS

D. APPLETON AND COMPANY
NEW YORK LONDON
1925

# PUBLISHERS' NOTE

Since the publication of the Gynecological and Obstetrical Monographs, definite advances have been made in some fields, while in others time has only served to modify, more or less definitely, views and practices heretofore held.

Such changes are inevitable and altogether desirable. Progress is reflected, whether in the form of new additional features or in the discard of the old.

The authors of the various monographs have, at the request of the publishers, furnished the material which brings the subject matter of each volume of the series down to the present. The material is presented to the profession in this supplemental volume.

# CONTENTS

# ILLUSTRATIONS

## MENSTRUATION AND ITS DISORDERS



## EXTRA-UTERINE PREGNANCY



## GYNECOLOGICAL AND OBSTETRICAL PATHOLOGY



## PELVIC NEOPLASMS



## SYMPTOMS GYNECOLOGICAL

# PELVIC INFLAMMATION IN WOMEN

JOHN OSBORN POLAK, M.D.

## APPENDIX

Since the completion of this monograph in 1922 much has been added to the literature of obstetrics and gynecology; yet there have been practically no contributions to the pathology, the diagnosis, or clinical course of pelvic inflammation.

This is not true however in regard to treatment, and I am pleased to note that the therapeutics and operative procedures of the dual specialty employed in many of the larger clinics—particularly in those that are under the direction of a single chief—have become more standardized. This we believe to be the result of a better appreciation of the pathology and the inflammatory tissue reaction which takes place when the organism is inoculated by pyogenic bacteria and a better understanding of the subject of immunity; for in the final analysis, the only reason why any woman recovers from an infection is that she produces within herself an immunity against it. This fact cannot be too much stressed nor be too often repeated; hence as a corollary to this fact, it may be stated that conditions like toxemia, hemorrhage, trauma, exhaustion, or operative shock, which temporarily or permanently reduce the individual resistance, afford a more favorable soil for the development of infection.

Other fundamental facts in the etiology and development of infection are an avenue of entrance and the life history and characteristics of the organism which is introduced at the time of inoculation. Thus in the treatment of gonorrheal vagititis, the fact that the gonococcus *must have moisture in which to live—and dies in a dry atmosphere*—is the basis for the so-called "dry treatment" the technic of which is as follows: After the active symptoms have subsided under the employment of postural care and cleanliness, the patient is placed in the Sims' or in the knee-chest position and the perineum retracted with a Sims' speculum. This allows the entrance of air and balloons the vagina. The vaginal mucosa is then dried with pledgets of sterilized cotton and the mucous membrane is thoroughly exposed to hot dry air from an electric drier, or from a dentist's bulb, the cannula of which has been flamed in an alcohol lamp. When the vaginal lining is thoroughly dried, bismuth subcarbonate is blown over the surface with a powder blower, this coats the mucosa with a bland non-irritating substance. This technic is repeated daily. Clinically the results have been most satisfactory.

**Endocervicitis.**—Time and experience are throwing new light on the far-reaching results of endocervicitis. The importance of endocervicitis in the causation of abortion cannot be underestimated; neither can we ignore its significance as the forerunner of cervical cancer or its effect on the functional activity of the ovary. Hence it is apparent that endocervicitis must be cured.

Several new suggestions have been offered and are being tried out. With the introduction of mercurochrome into gynecology it is but natural that it should be used in the treatment of endocervicitis.

It is a well-known clinical fact that infection of any type, however insignificant, leaves its mark upon the organ or tissue involved; therefore it is apparent that the shorter the duration and the more limited the area of reaction, the less permanent is the pathology that will remain. This is certainly true in cervical infection; for in the case of the superficial erosion with its overgrowth of lymphoid tissue which does not involve the gland elements of the endocervix, the disease is readily cured. On the other hand, infection of the cervical endometrium with extension of the infective process into the racemose structures of the cervical glands excites a tissue reaction in the periglandular structures which permanently increases the bulk of the cervix and spreads to the lymphatics of the parametrium and perimetrium.

With these facts in mind it is desirable to cure endocervicitis before its chronicity is established. Frank suggests in subacute endocervicitis, that after the superficial mucus has been cleared away with the peroxid paste referred to in the chapter on endocervicitis, small wooden (destructible) applicators wrapped with sterile cotton, be wet with a 2 per cent solution of mercurochrome and placed side by side in the cervical canal, until they exert some pressure on the mucosa. This tends to evacuate the mucous content from the superficial glands, and permits the mercurochrome to penetrate into the adjacent tissue. This treatment may be repeated every second or third day.

J. V. D. Young treats endocervicitis by aspiration, using specially designed glass tubes which fit over the vaginal portio and are attached to a suction pump which by producing a vacuum causes a passive hyperemia in the cervix. Aspiration empties the cervical glands of their contained mucus and thus establishes drainage. We have preceded this procedure with multiple puncture of the portio which allows the withdrawal of blood by suction and further depletes the cervix. Suction for ten minutes empties the cervical glands, diminishes the size of the cervix, the tenderness of the parametria, and the amount of the cervical discharge. When the apparatus is removed and the blood and mucus have been swabbed away with sterile cotton, the portio and canal are painted over with a 2 per cent mercurochrome solution. This procedure should be repeated twice a week. The clinical results in selected cases have been all that the originator claimed.

Graves and Pemberton are employing deep crucial cauterization of the cervix under anesthesia.

In cases of ectropion with coincident erosion without tissue loss the technic consists of drawing the cervix down, protecting the introitus and vaginal walls with the proper specula and then with a heavy flat cautery knife, at dull red heat, making four linear incisions through the cervical mucosa from just below the internal os to the vaginal portio. Contraction of these scars inverts the external os, heals the erosion and cures the discharge.

The author, at the suggestion of Gibson, has employed circular cauterization of the everted, eroded area, using a heavy flat-tipped blade, carefully destroying the entire mucosa for a distance of two centimeters up the canal. The cosmetic as well as the subjective result in these patients is all that can be desired.

It was feared that such extensive use of the cautery, like in the injudicious employment of radium within the cervix, might be followed by cervical stenosis and produce dystocia during labor.

A review of our follow-up work on a sufficient number of cases which include a large percentage of pregnancies and labors, shows that the contour of the cervix has been restored, the erosion cured and that the scar tissue has in no way interfered with course of pregnancy or labor.

We are convinced that *too many operations are being done on the cervix in child-bearing women.* Extensive excision and amputation should be reserved for the chronic infections with marked cystic formation, hypertrophy, and deep multiple lacerations. Plastics and trachelo-plasty should be deferred until the woman has completed her child-bearing period.

**Salpingitis.**—*No case of acute salpingitis needs operation:* time and supportive treatment are the fundamental principles in the management of pelvic inflammation; for it is the adaptability of the normal organism which produces the resistance to infection and renders the living or non-living invader innocuous. By one means or another the harmful agent whether it be the organism or its toxin must be metabolized, digested, destroyed, detoxicated, or excreted. To accomplish this means increased tissue function, increase in the red and white cell resistance, increased metabolism, with more oxygen and greater oxygen carrying power. The leukocyte is the direct enemy of all pyogenic bacteria; hence the value of a leukocyte and polymorphonuclear reaction in any infection.

Recent work by Schmitt and Gellhorn in gonorrhea with milk injection seems to show that the introduction into the system of a non-specific protein will increase the leukocyte reaction and cause the absorption of exudates, the absorption of abscesses and the disappearance of pus tubes of gonorrheal origin. As is the case with all protein therapy, it should be employed as early as possible in the course of the disease in order to be efficacious; for the earlier the cell reaction is excited the less chance the bacteria have to multiply.

At Gellhorn's suggestion, we have been using milk, ordinary warm, unboiled hospital milk, in our clinic for something over two years; and while I can frankly say that we have not seen the clinical miracles reported by its sponsors—such as an "abscess with definite fluctuation disappear"—we have seen exudates melt away, enlarged tubal masses disappear and the patient generally improve.

One good point about milk injections is that their employment does no harm even if the injection does no good. The anaphylaxis is mild if it occurs at all. This is not so when sera have been employed. The intramuscular use of milk provokes a leukocytic reaction, which is at its height about four hours after the injection and gradually falls during the succeeding twenty-four hours. The reaction is more marked and the results more convincing when the gonococcus is the offending organism than in infections by bacteria of higher virulence.

In the early stages of gonorrheal salpingitis, and in parametritic exudates of both postpartum and postoperative origin, it is our custom to begin the injections of milk as soon as the diagnosis has been arrived at. We usually begin with 5 c.c. injected intramuscularly every second day. If there is no reaction, the quantity is increased to 10 c.c. The technic is simple. After the usual iodin preparation of the skin the injection is made into muscle structures just below the crest of the ilium. Aside from the local reaction at the site of the injection, the well-being of the patient is generally improved, and she is promptly relieved of pain.

A study of the circulation of the uterus shows that the interior with its endometrial lining has but a poor blood supply. This is made up of terminal arterioles and venous radicals which are shut off from the abundant circulation of the outer coat by the firm contraction of the uterus. The more perfect the contraction and retraction of the uterus, the more intense is the passive hyperemia and the isolation of the endometrial tissues; hence it will be seen that the empty contracted uterus is the greatest safeguard against infections of endometrial origin.

The majority of parametrial inflammations spread from cervix tears or from cervix infection and develop reactions in the form of exudates in the cellular structures adjacent to the cervix. *These exudates are protective* and may be considered as favorable to the prognosis. Their absorption may be hastened by the use of small blood transfusions, intramuscular injections of milk, diathermy, and the daily use of the "sun" rays. But *rest* and *time dissolve all exudates.*

**Blood Transfusions.**—In thrombophlebitis and bacteriemia, the bacteria are in the blood stream; in the former they are within the clot multiplying and producing liquefaction until they are set free into the blood stream; in the latter, the bacteria are circulating in the blood, and rapidly multiply, for blood is an ideal culture medium and furnishes the necessary heat for growth and development; hence the longer the infection exists, the greater is the bacterial multiplication and the greater number of colonies will be found on culture. This fact emphasizes the necessity for early treatment.

Since the publication of our original article, we have been constantly using direct transfusion of blood in infection and have made some clinical observations worthy of note:

(1) *Each case must not only be typed but must be matched,* the matching should be done immediately before giving the transfusion; for infection seems to exert some biochemical change in the cells and serum, which may produce severe reaction in the recipient unless this care is taken.

(2) The transfusion should be given when the temperature is down or during a remission. This is particulaurly important in thrombophlebitis.

(3) Direct transfusion is most satisfactory. The use of the citrate method has been entirely given up in our practice and is replaced by the Unger method which is simple and easily done.

Direct transfusion of perfectly matched blood increases the blood-pressure, slows the heart's action, stimulates the defensive cell reaction and generally improves the function of the several viscera. Our experience shows that the clinical benefits are apparent for three or four days, during this time, the appearance of the patient improves, the pulse becomes slower and the temperature shows greater remissions. The transfusion should be repeated on the fourth day. Quantities of over 400 c.c. do not give the result that transfusions of 250 or 300 c.c. can be expected to give. It is well to precede the operation with a hypodermic of morphin

¼ grn., scopolanin $\frac{1}{130}$ grn., which insures passivity on the part of the woman.

**Mercurochrome.**—Piper, in the clinic of Professor Hirst at the University Hospital in Philadelphia, began his experimental work as early as 1919 with the intravenous injections of solutions of mercurochrome. Later Hugh Young, of Baltimore, advocated its use in streptococcic bacteriemia. Piper demonstrated that a solution of mercurochrome (5 Gms. per kilo of body weight) introduced in the blood stream of a patient with a streptococcic bacteriemia would sterilize the blood in the course of a few hours and do this without more serious injury to the human organism than a temporary diminution in the urinary output and the production of a diarrhea. To arrive at a safe dosage, one that would kill the bacteria, yet produce no marked general reaction, has been a difficult task.

According to Piper, severely ill patients are given intravenous injections of mercurochrome (5 Gm. per kilo of body weight). In all cases the urine was typical of any severe infection and the mercurochrome did not change the blood in any way, except that the leukocytes were somewhat increased in some instances. A definite reaction, however, routinely followed the injection (no benefit was observed unless the reaction was severe). Within the first hour vomiting frequently occurred; in less than two hours there was a definite diarrhea, and within the first six hours a marked chill with a rise of temperature up to 105° F. took place. Following this there was a gradual fall in the temperature with a proportionate decrease in the pulse rate until the temperature reached subnormal and then the temperature gradually rose to normal or slightly above. The diarrhea continued over a day or two. The solution must be absolutely fresh and clear. The injection should be made very slowly with the temperature of the solution as near 100° F. as possible. Subsequent injections of the drug may be given, but the author has never repeated the dose so long as there was a trace of the dye in the urine or feces. Puerperal septicemia is so serious and so frequently fatal that heroic measures are justified.

Fifty c.c. of 1 per cent solution of neutral acriflavin has also been employed for its antibactericidal powers and has been used intravenously for bacteriemia. It is, however, less effective than mercurochrome.

Both from experimental and clinical observation it can be stated *that these dyes should not be used for sterilization of the blood except where there is a positive blood culture.* This entails waiting for the bacteriological report and waiting is dangerous in sepsis, if the bacteria have reached the blood stream. Hence, it has been our practice as soon as a presumptive diagnosis of blood stream infection is made, to take a blood *culture at the same time that we transfuse our patient,* and if the *culture comes back positive* and the patient has not shown the usual improvement from transfusion mercurochrome is used intravenously, following the technic of Piper.

**Antistreptococcus Serum in Sepsis.**—Through the work of H. C. Bailey at the Bellevue Maternity Hospital, New York, antistreptococcus serum has received renewed recognition. Bailey studied a small series of cases in which the uterine culture showed the Streptococcus hæmolyticus but the blood cultures were negative. He used from 50 to 100 c.c. of the serum in twenty-four hours. In all, 13 cases were treated, with a mortality of 15.3 per cent. It is difficult to deduce from this series what *real effect the serum had;* for we only know that on the fourth or fifth day post partum the interior of the uterus is infested with bacteria and we have many times on intra-uterine culture following labor or abortion recovered a hemolytic streptococcus, when the patient has been perfectly well and afebrile. Hence we feel that Bailey's results could be duplicated any time by leaving the patient alone. Serum, however, has a place in sepsis that is not generally recognized by the clinician and *that is for immunization.* If diphtheria, tetanus, typhoid, and other bacteral infections can be controlled by serum injections, it is reasonable to believe that similar results may be obtained in postpartum and postabortal infections. All infections excite hyperemia, exudation, cell migration, and proliferation. These processes vary with the virulence of the invader and the individual's adaptable resistance. Hence, anything that can sensitize the individual to infectious bacteria will diminish the severity of the attack. We have found an excellent use for serum as a preventive measure. Given a woman who is potentially infected, as for example, a craniotomy which has followed several unsuccessful attempts at delivery with forceps, or a woman with a history of having had repeated vaginal examinations through an unprepared vulva, with a temperature of 101° at the time of delivery; surely it may be presumed that such a patient will develop fever. Under these conditions 50 c.c. of the serum may be administered daily and the woman will become so immunized that the infection will be checked. *Serum is a preventive of sepsis, not a cure for it.* For according to serologists, after incubation and bacterial multiplication have taken place serum therapy is untenable.

# MENSTRUATION AND ITS DISORDERS

EMIL NOVAK, M.D.

## APPENDIX

In selecting for presentation in this supplementary chapter the more important contributions which have been made during the past two or three years in our knowledge of the general subject matter of this volume, an effort will be made to follow somewhat the same sequence as in the preceding chapters. In this way the reader can readily correlate any of the original chapters with the subjects treated in the present supplement. It may be added that only such matters have been included as might be expected to have an effect on the general complexion of the volume. An exhaustive review of the literature for even the past few years would scarcely be possible within the limits of even a very long chapter.

**Periodic Sexual Phenomena in the Lower Animals.**—Much of our knowledge of the physiology of menstruation has come, and more will undoubtedly come in the future, from the study of the corresponding process in the lower animals. Such investigations are being carried out by many investigators, and two or three contributions may be mentioned as especially important. The method suggested by Stockard and Papanicalou in 1917, whereby the stages of the sexual cycle can be so easily and so accurately determined by the study of vaginal smears, has proved to be of inestimable value and has come into quite general use. The original demonstration was made upon guinea-pigs, but since then other investigators have extended the observation to a number of other laboratory animals. The value of such a simple method of study is apparent when one bears in mind that in most of these animals there are practically no signs of œstrus to be seen in the external genitalia.

The recent contributions of Allen, Doisy, and their coworkers upon the hormone of the ovarian follicle have excited much interest. They find that the subcutaneous injection of liquor folliculi and extracts of the ovarian follicles of swine brings about in spayed mice changes exactly similar to those of œstrus. They report experiments which would indicate that the follicular hormone is responsible for œstrous growth and secretion, sex instinct, and the attainment of puberty. They were unable to confirm the results of Herrmann, who had previously reported somewhat similar results from the lipoid principles prepared from the corpus luteum. The investigations of Allen and Doisy are extremely suggestive, although it is too soon to conclude that the follicular hormone is the all-important element produced by the ovary. This matter is further discussed in the paragraph on The Ovarian Factor Concerned in Menstruation.

**Is There a Loss of Uterine Mucosa at the Time of Menstruation?**—Since the writing of this monograph, the author has undergone a decided change of opinion with regard to the changes occurring in the endometrium during menstruation. The postmenstrual, interval, and premenstrual char-

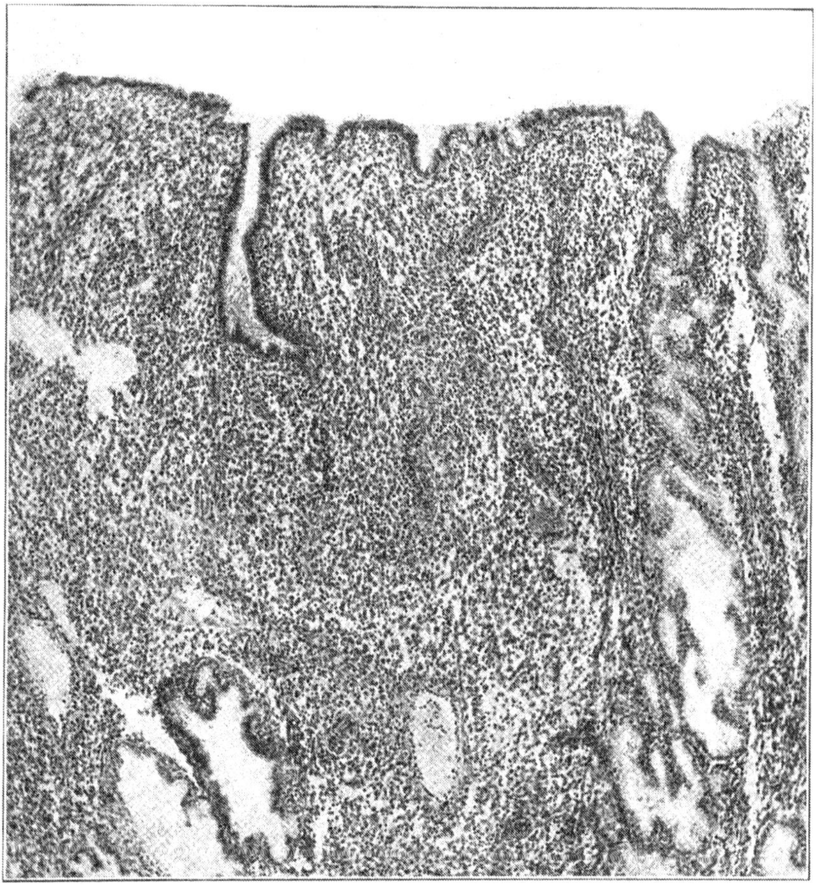

FIG. 1.—ENDOMETRIUM JUST BEFORE MENSTRUATION, taken from a patient about to menstruate, but not yet bleeding at time of operation.

The dilated tortuous glands, the intact surface epithelium and the marked infiltration of the lymphocytes and polymorphonuclears may be seen.

acteristics of the endometrium are quite well established, but there has in the past been much difference of opinion as to the changes occurring during the bleeding phase. This applies especially to the question of whether or not any considerable portion of the uterine mucosa is lost at this time. Schröder's view that there is an extensive casting off of the mucosa during menstruation has never obtained general acceptance in this country, as one may learn by a glance through even the recent editions of our text-books on gynecology and obstetrics. A recent study by the author, in association with

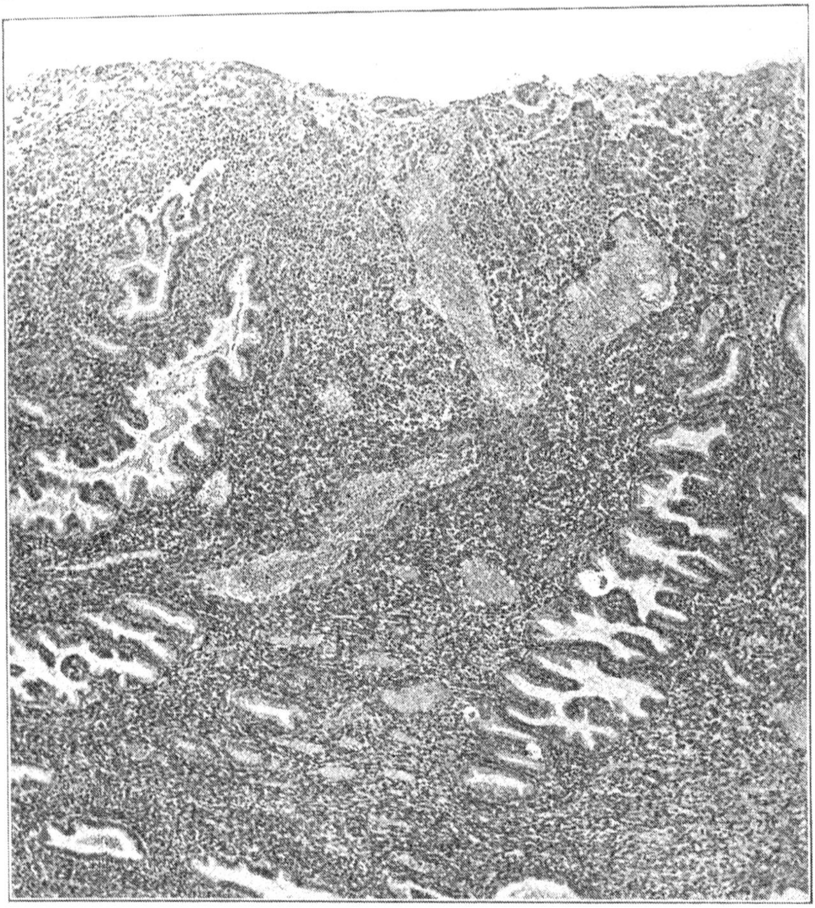

FIG. 2.—ENDOMETRIUM ON THE FIRST DAY OF MENSTRUATION, showing the compacta, spongiosa, and part of the basalis.

The greatly dilated blood vessels, some of which are opening directly on the surface (rhexis), are especially prominent. There is a marked infiltration, especially of the compacta, the upper portion of which is being cast off in small particles. There are considerable individual differences in the degree of this endometrial loss on the first day.

TeLinde, has convinced us that there is characteristically a definite loss of tissue at menstruation. Our findings may be summarized as follows:

Our material consisted of twelve uteri removed during some phase of actual menstruation, together with a number removed immediately before or just after menstruation. The study of this material, by methods which we believe eliminated errors of technic, convinced us that extensive loss of tissue is the rule during menstruation. The entire superficial or compact layer, as well as most of the deeper or spongy layer, is thrown off. It is possible that there may be exceptions to this, but we have not observed them. On the first day the surface of the mucosa may be quite intact, but more commonly it shows beginning loss of tissue. By the second day the throw-

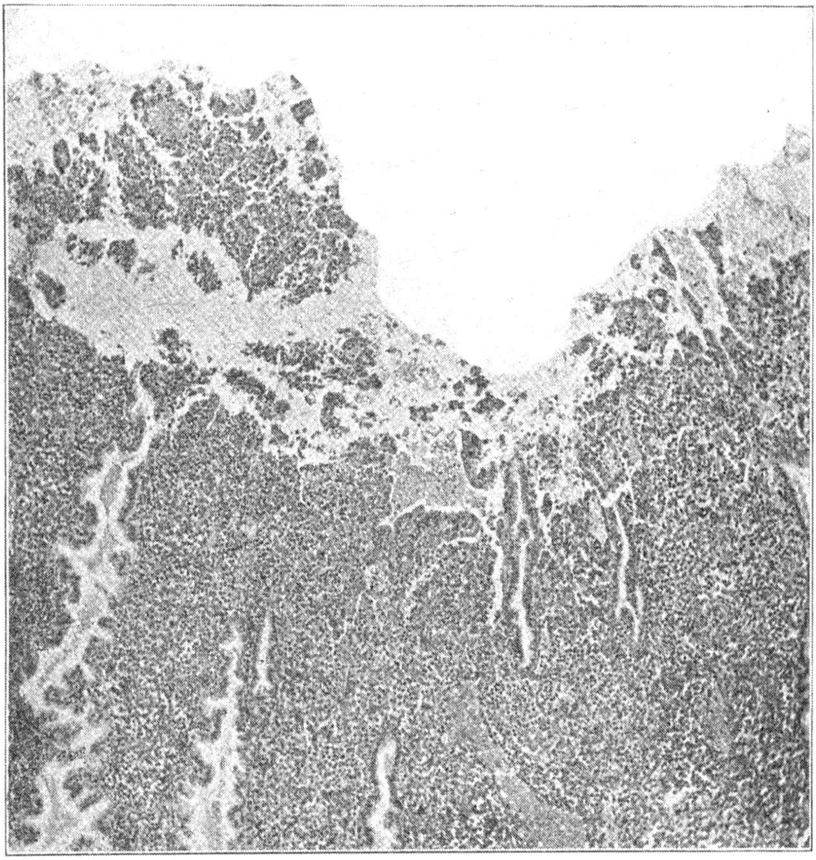

FIG. 3.—SECTION OF ANOTHER PORTION OF THE SURFACE OF THE ENDOMETRIUM OF THE UTERUS SHOWN IN FIG. 2, illustrating the crumbling away of the compacta and the marked cellular infiltration (slightly higher power).

ing off has become very extensive, all the compacta and most of the spongiosa being gone. Regeneration changes are usually evident on the third day, and may be quite marked.

The desquamation of mucosa is preceded by extensive infiltration with polymorphonuclear leukocytes, this infiltration being marked for a short time before the actual clinical onset of menstruation. The throwing off of the mucosa does not commonly occur as an extensive shedding in large masses. It is a sort of crumbling, molecular process, small strips and bits of granular degenerated mucosa being cast off until only the basalis, and perhaps a few spongiosal rests, are left. The desquamated endometrial portions may be recovered from the menstrual discharge, as we were able to show. Pyknotic changes are prominent at the beginning of menstruation.

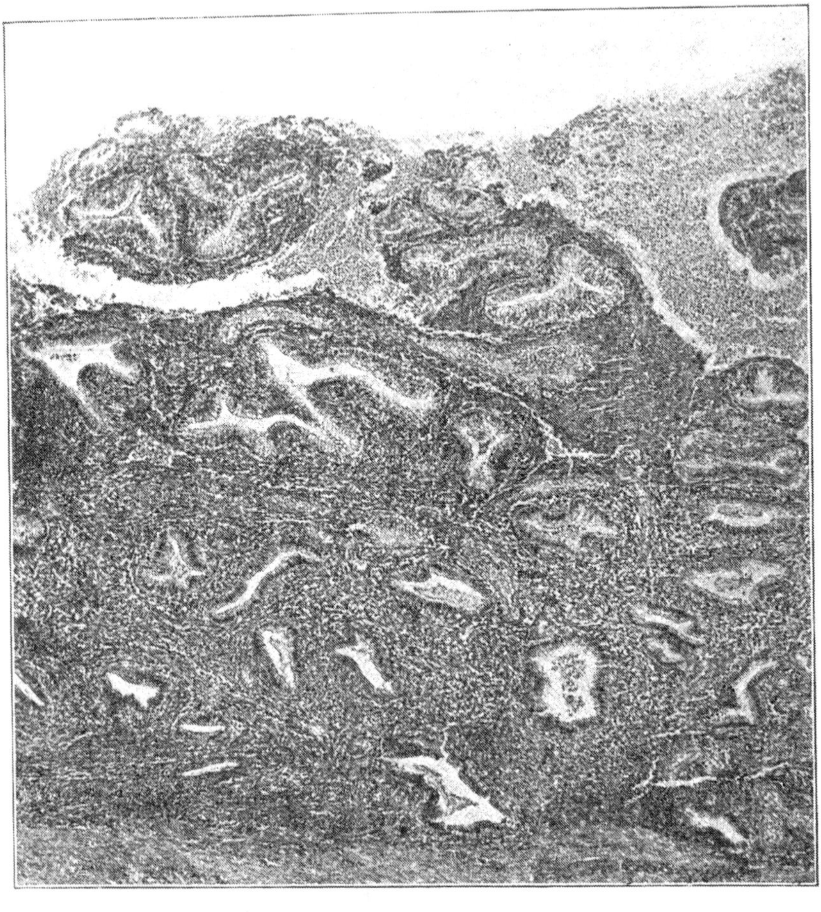

FIG. 4.—ENDOMETRIUM ON SECOND DAY OF MENSTRUATION, showing the basalis with only a small part of the spongiosa intact.
The compacta and the greater part of the spongiosa have been cast off.

Regeneration is remarkably rapid, especially the epithelization of the surface. The source of the new epithelium is chiefly the epithelium of the basal stumps of the uterine glands. Strange to say, mitoses are not very frequent, appearing in largest number when the epithelial layer is already complete.

While diapedesis may perhaps play some part in the mechanism of the menstrual bleeding, rhexis is certainly the most important factor. It can be demonstrated histologically, although its occurrence is self-evident, in view of the extensive tissue loss associated with menstruation.

**The Ovarian Factor Concerned in Menstruation.**—The generally accepted view is still that the corpus luteum is the ovarian constituent which is most directly concerned with the occurrence of menstruation. There is

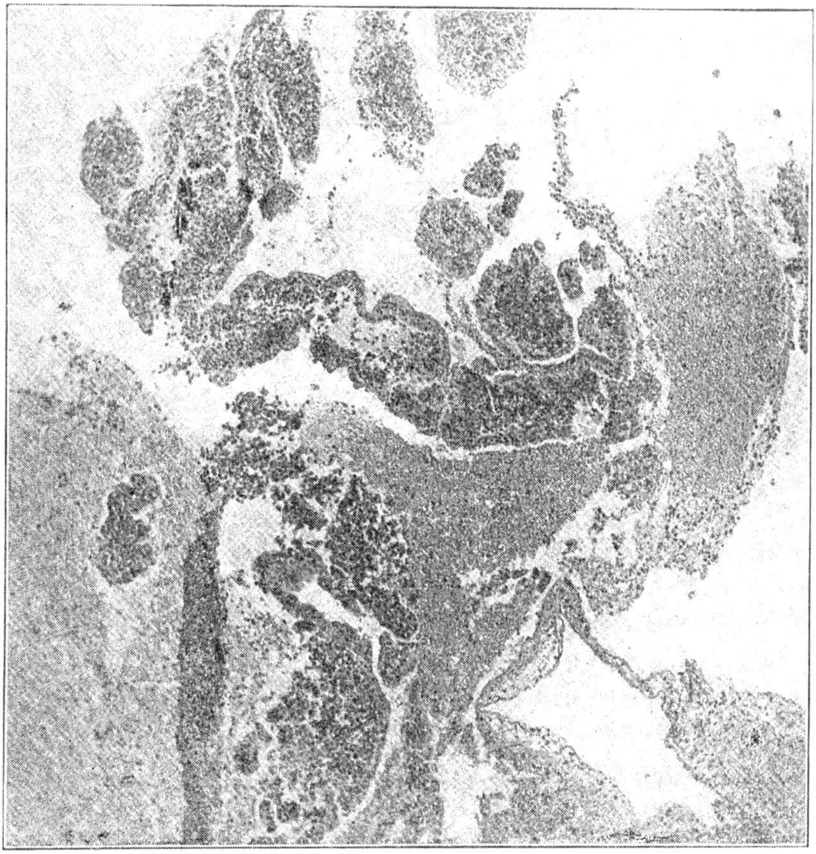

Fig. 5.—Blood Clot Obtained from Cavity of the Menstruating Uterus Whose Endometrium Is Shown in Fig. 4.

Cast-off particles of the upper two layers of the endometrium are seen, including not only surface epithelium, but also considerable stroma and numerous glands.

considerable confusion, however, as to just how this influence is exerted. Certainly the corpus luteum has nothing to do with the production of the actual menstrual bleeding itself. It has much to do, however, with the remarkable hypertrophic premenstrual or pregravid changes seen in the mucosa just before the appearance of the bleeding. These premenstrual changes are a *sine qua non* to menstruation, for the stage of actual menstrual bleeding consists in a transition from this high point of development to the low point observed just after menstruation. This transition phase is accompanied, as previously described, with the loss of the upper endometrial layers. Clinically it is accompanied by the bleeding which we call menstruation. The actual initiation of the bleeding, however, is due not to the

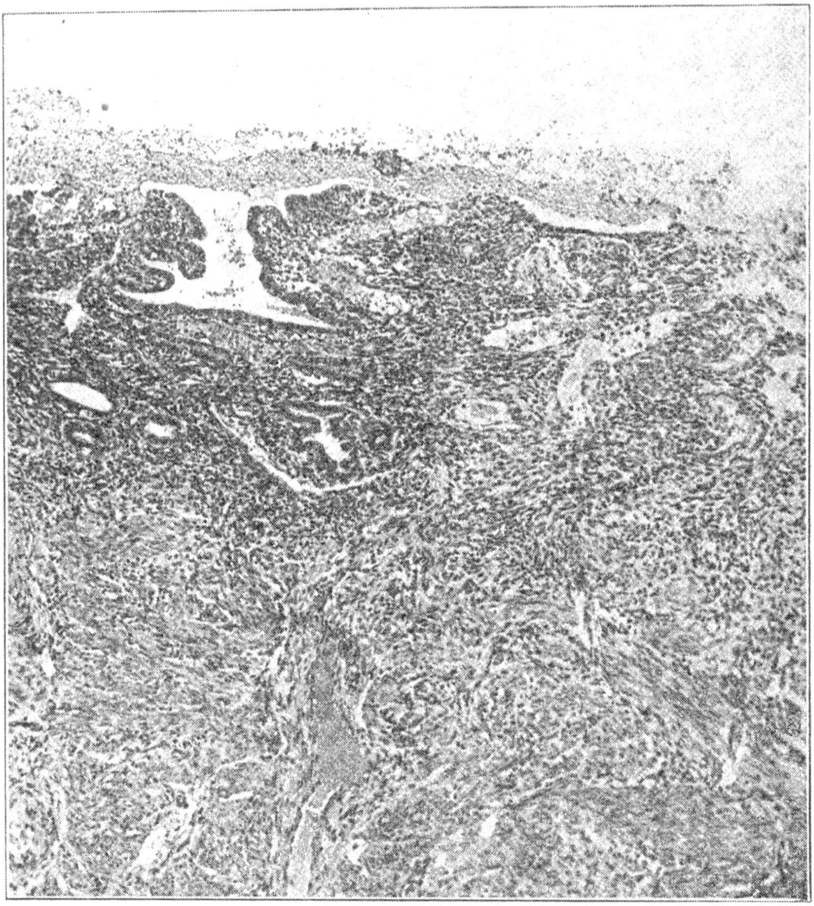

FIG. 6.—ENDOMETRIUM ON THE THIRD DAY OF MENSTRUATION, showing practically only the basalis left intact.

The epithelization of the surface has already begun, by the outgrowth of epithelium along the surface from the remaining glands.

corpus luteum, but to some other factor, probably the death of the ovum thrown off from the ovary something like two weeks previously.

Another factor which must be considered is the probable participation in the menstrual mechanism of the ovarian follicle. Marshall and others have stressed this very strongly in previous years, and more recently the investigations of Allen and Doisy have called renewed attention to the subject. As detailed in a previous paragraph, these authors have been able by the subcutaneous injection of liquor folliculi obtained from swine to bring about in mice changes which are in every way similar to those seen during normal œstrus. They believe that the follicular hormone is the "principal female sex hormone," and that it is responsible for the changes of œstrus, the sex instincts of the female, and the changes of puberty. The probabilities are, of course, that the ovary is an organ of multiple and interlocking endocrine function, and that the ovum itself, the follicles, and the corpus luteum all play a part in the mechanism of menstruation. Much remains to be learned as to the part played by each factor, and as to the manner in which their rôles dovetail into one another.

**A Menstrual Toxin (Menotoxin).**—Chapter I is devoted to a consideration of superstitions based on the belief that the menstruating woman is a source of danger to herself and those about her. Ridiculous though many of these have seemed, a degree of confirmation is given them by the recent observations of Schick, corroborated later by Macht and Lubin. Schick observed that cut flowers handled by women who happened to be menstruating quickly withered. By extending these observations he concluded that the skin secretion of menstruating women contains some toxic substance which exerts this unfavorable effect upon flowers. For example, this effect could be avoided if the woman wore sterile gloves in handling the flowers. Macht and Lubin, studying the effect of various body fluids and secretions upon the growth of seedlings, concluded that a toxic substance (menotoxin) is found in the blood serum, blood corpuscles, saliva, sweat, milk, and other secretions of practically every menstruating woman, although there are marked individual variations in the degree of toxic action. The most marked effects are seen just before the beginning of the periods, and during the first few days of the flow. They suggest that the menstrual toxin is related chemically to oxycholesterin. Very recently Labhardt has reported observations discrediting those of Schick, so that further confirmation along these lines seems necessary. It should, moreover, be borne in mind that the observations of Schick, and the later ones of Macht and Lubin, indicate only that certain of the body fluids of menstruating women contain a substance or substances injurious to plant life, and that they cannot, of course, be interpreted as indicating that menstruation is a cleansing process. Their greatest practical bearing, it would seem, lies in the fact that they indicate a more or less systemic reaction to the menstrual phenomenon.

**Metabolic Changes During Menstruation.**—A recent study by Wakeham indicates that there is a fall in *basal metabolism* during or immediately after menstruation, and that there is a premenstrual rise. He further suggests, tentatively, that (1) basal metabolism is considerably higher, on the average, in those engaged in strenuous labor than in those of sedentary occupations; (2) that basal metabolism fluctuations in those living under uniform conditions is less than in those whose mode of life is more varied; (3) that the basal metabolism variation due to the menstrual cycle, while in every case less than the average daily fluctuations, is greater in active women than in sedentary women; (4) that causes which produce too frequent menstruation are likely to be accompanied by high basal metabolism; (5) that causes which delay or suppress menstruation are likely to be accompanied by low basal metabolism.

The *blood calcium,* according to a study of the ash of the blood from twenty women through two or three menstrual periods, varies between wide limits, but a tendency to rise with menstruation was noted, in 57 per cent. In 14 per cent the calcium content dropped.

The *sugar metabolism* of menstruating women was studied by Heilig, who gave women 100 Gm. of saccharose on the first and second day of menstruation. The majority reacted with a marked hyperglycemia and a subsequent glycosuria.

Recent studies by Bond would indicate that there is a relation between the *ammonia coefficient* and menstruation. In the postmenstrual and intermenstrual periods the coefficient varies little from the intermenstrual average, but during the seven days previous to the period—*i.e.,* the premenstrual period—there is a marked rise. This rise appears to be due to a rise in the total output of urinary ammonia rather than to a decrease in the total output of urinary nitrogen.

**Blood-Pressure During Menstruation.**—Amos finds in a recent study of the subject that there is a decided fall of blood-pressure early in the menstrual period, and that this is often preceded, a day or so before the commencement of the period, by a rise, and further, that after the rather sudden fall, there is again a rise toward the end of menstruation, or a day or so after the period has finished.

**Unsatisfactory Results from Benzyl Benzoate in Dysmenorrhea.**—A recent report by the Council on Pharmacy and Chemistry of the American Medical Association calls attention to the generally disappointing results obtained from benzyl compounds, particularly the benzoate and the acetate, in the treatment of many conditions for which they had been highly vaunted. A recent paper by Gruber and Shackleford deals with the same subject. Certainly these views correspond with my own experience with the drug in the treatment of primary dysmenorrhea. The results, in my own hands, have been practically worthless, certainly not to be compared with those obtained from atropin, fallible though the latter is.

**Hyperplasia of the Endometrium.**—A recent study of 66 cases by Novak and Martzloff has served to emphasize the importance of this condition, already described on page 246 of this monograph. The lesion was first described by Cullen as far back as 1900. Clinically, its characteristic symptom is bleeding, while pathologically it is characterized by hyperplasia of both epithelial and stromal elements in varying degree and in varying proportion. The glands are of the "swiss cheese" pattern, large dilated glands being found side by side with glands which are small and narrow. The epithelium is at times considerably thickened, while the stroma is often overabundant and may give evidence of proliferative activity by the presence of an unusual number of mitoses.

Grossly the endometrium may be enormously increased in amount and may present the polypoid picture which has so often been incorrectly described as "chronic polypoid endometritis." In almost half of our cases, however, it was of normal thickness, and in over one half it was smooth rather than polypoid. The hyperplasia may be localized in uterine polypi, in which case, unless associated with other lesions or with strangulation of the polyp, bleeding has not been a symptom. The hyperplasia pattern is not

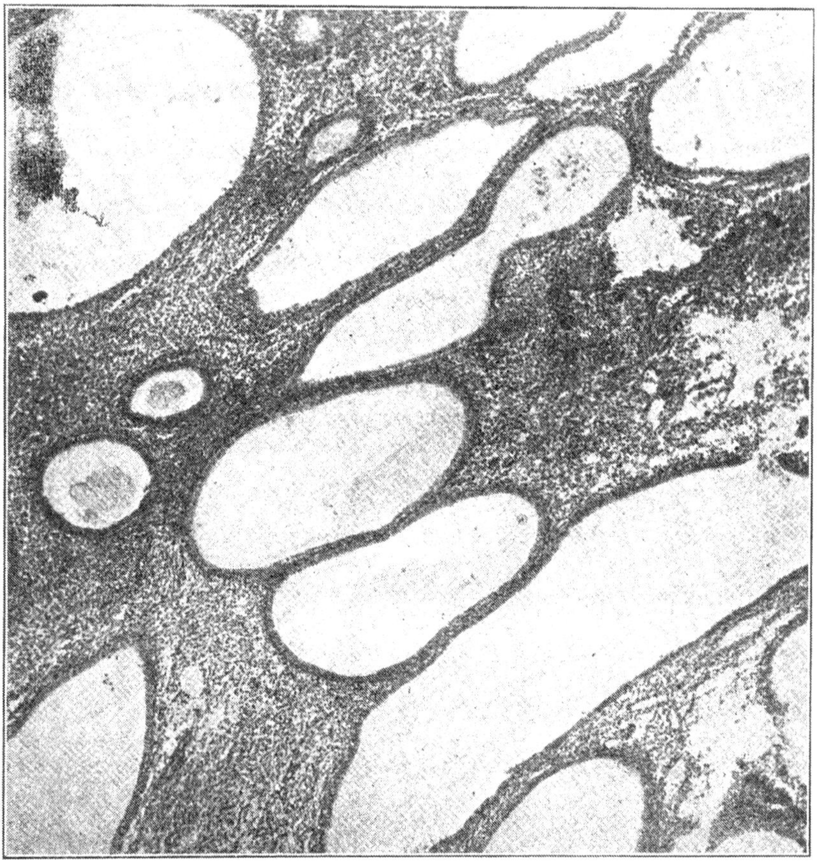

FIG. 7.—TYPICAL HYPERPLASIA OF MARKED DEGREE from a woman of 43, who had had uterine bleeding for several months.
Note the typical "swiss cheese" pattern of the glands.

uncommon with adenomyoma, in either the endometrium of the surface or that of the islets in the musculature.

About one half of our patients with hyperplasia were above 40 years of age while the remainder were women under the age of 40. The occurrence of hyperplasia in girls near the age of puberty is, in our experience, not common (less than 5 per cent). Our study shows no definite abnormality in the menstrual history of these patients prior to the onset of the symptoms of hyperplasia. With the onset of the symptoms of hyperplasia there was, however, in almost every case, excessive menstruation manifested usually by an increase in both the amount and duration of the menstrual discharge.

Menorrhagia or metrorrhagia may occur as symptoms of hyperplasia, the former being the more common of the two. The passage of blood clots is not unusual. Amenorrhea, as part of the symptom-complex of hyperplasia, was noted in about one sixth of our cases. Pregnancy occurring after the onset of hyperplasia is uncommon in our study, but did occur in two patients. About one half of our patients had had one or more full-term pregnancies prior to the onset of the symptoms which are associated with hyperplasia.

Schröder believes that an absence of corpora lutea in the ovaries is a characteristic finding with hyperplasia. We have found some exceptions to this rule, so that the matter needs further investigation. The characteristic gland pattern is attribued by some merely to epithelial hyperplasia, and by some to simple cystic distention, while to us the evidence suggests that an enormous overgrowth of the basal layer of the endometrium and an absence of the superficial functioning layers is sufficient to explain the characteristic picture.

The therapeutic measures to be considered for the relief of the uterine bleeding associated with hyperplasia are curettage, organotherapy, radiotherapy, and hysterectomy. There are probably a certain number of mild cases which get well spontaneously. Curettage is necessary to make a diagnosis and may bring about relief of symptoms. Recurrence of the bleeding within a comparatively short time is more common, and repeated curettage may be necessary in the case of young patients where both radiotherapy and hysterectomy are undesirable. At the menopausal age the bleeding can be checked by sufficient dosage of either x-ray or radium. Hysterectomy is reserved for intractable cases where radium is unavailable or where associated lesions make laparotomy preferable to simple abolition of the menstrual function.

The most important clinical group of hyperplasia cases, and the largest one, is that occurring at or near the menopausal age. The importance of the condition at this age lies in the fact that it is brought into diagnostic conflict with cancer. While it is still true that climacteric bleeding should be looked upon as of cancerous causation until this assumption is disproved the fact remains that in many cases the cause will be revealed as hyperplasia, a benign condition with no tendency toward malignancy. This is an important point to impress upon those interested in educating the laity in the early recognition of cancer, for there can be no doubt that not a few women with climacteric bleeding delay seeking medical advice through dread of being told that cancer is the cause of their symptoms. Any element of justifiable hopefulness that can be injected into the situation will be of material aid in the cancer education of the public.

**The Cause of the Vaginal Bleeding of Tubal Pregnancy.**—The studies of Sampson, in 1913, led him to the conclusion that the external bleeding of tubal pregnancy has its source in the endometrium. A similar view has been recently expressed by Polak and Wolfe, although these authors believe that in at least a certain number of cases, more particularly those of the interstitial type, the hemorrhage may proceed from the placental site itself. Novak and Darner, in a recent study, find that the bleeding in these cases is characteristically initiated by the death of the embryo, although other factors, probably of hormone nature, are undoubtedly concerned in its frequent continuance for many weeks. The source of these factors is probably in some unknown way associated with the persistence of trophoblastic elements in the tubal wall long after the actual death of the embryo. In cases of tubal pregnancy in which the fetus is still alive, amenorrhea is the rule instead of bleeding. Cases of this type of course are far less numerous than those of the bleeding type, in which the fetus has succumbed.

**Organotherapy in Functional Hemorrhages.**—In the hemorrhages of puberty, Stickel and Zondek got successful results from the use of pituitary and testicular extracts, but met with failure from the use of corpus luteum and thyroid extracts. Twelve of fifteen patients in this group were cured by the organotherapy, while three were failures. In hemorrhages occurring between the ages of 20 and 40, corpus luteum was more successful, although the best results were obtained from pineal, pituitary, and testicular extracts. Of this group, organ extracts were of little or no value. The authors assume that many women at this age show a definite arteriosclerosis, and they suggest the injection of a mixture of pituitary and testicular extracts.

**Calcium Treatment of Menopausal Hemorrhages.**—A study by Hornung was undertaken with the idea that perhaps climacteric functional hemorrhages were associated with a disturbance of the coagulation mechanism as a a result of the disturbed function of the ovary. He states that in 80 per cent of the cases the intravenous injection of 10 c.c. of a 10 per cent solution of calcium chlorid brought about a cessation of the hemorrhages, though in some cases a second injection was necessary. He reports failure in only 8 per cent of the cases.

**Vicarious Menstruation.**—A rather extensive study of this somewhat confused subject was made by Roth, who found 225 cases recorded since 1870. In 30 per cent the vicarious bleeding took place from the nose; in 10 per cent from the skin or from fistulas; in 8 per cent from the lungs; in 4 or 5 per cent each from the breast, stomach, mouth, and throat; in 3.5 to 4.5 per cent from the bladder, ear, eye, intestine, larynx, trachea, kidneys, and vagina. In 25 per cent the bleeding was purely vicarious, in 75 per cent it was supplementary to the normal flow. Three fatal cases occurred, the vicarious hemorrhages coming from the lungs or bronchi. Roth emphasizes the fact that only cases of the more severe types are published, so that the phenomenon is probably more common than might be surmised from the literature. He mentions two personally observed cases. In one the patient began to bleed from the bowel at regular intervals nine months after the onset of the menopause. In the other, the blood was vomited, without retching, at each menstrual period. At all other times the stomach was free from blood.

**Transplantation of the Ovaries.**—A number of reports dealing with this subject have appeared within the past few years. Tuffier has described a method of autotransplantation of the ovary with its pedicle within the uterus. The operation is said by him to be followed not only by the preservation of menstruation, but also by the possibility of impregnation. The study of 98 cases by Bell leads him to advocate ovarian grafting very strongly in suitable cases, although it cannot be compared with preservation of the natural connections of the ovary. Sippel's report, based on 57 cases, includes a discussion of the employment of transplantation of the ovaries in such conditions as infantilism, premature and artificial menopause, and premature senility. Finally, attention may be called to the recent review of this subject by Martin, the sixth which this author has published. His conclusions are as follows: (1) Clinically there is very little to encourage one to believe that transplantation of the ovaries as practiced up to the present time has more than speculative value as a surgical procedure. (2) There is some evidence that autotransplants are of some value in deferring the symptoms of the menopause and delaying the cessation of menstruation. It is difficult, however, not to attribute some of this evidence to suggestive therapeutics or to unattached ovarian tissue left in situ. (3) There is practically no convincing evidence that homotransplants have been successful in the human female. (4) There is no evidence that heterotransplants have been successful where the human female has been the recipient. (5) There is some encouraging evidence recorded in experimental animal surgery that not only autotransplants, but homotransplants and even heterotransplants have been successful and the sexual function of the castrated animal maintained. (6) The technic followed by the various operators on human females, in too many instances, seems unsurgical and too often is incompletely and loosely recorded, leaving the impression that the conclusions derived from such work must be unreliable. (7) There is, however, encouraging evidence in all of this endeavor to lead one to hope that the subject will be pursued experimentally, especially for the purpose of devising a rational and simple technic, based on the work of the serologists, the endocrinologists, the hematologists, and the practical clinical surgeons.

**Growth of Human Ovarian Tissue in Vitro.**—Zondek and Wolff report the results of experiments upon the cultivation of human ovarian tissue outside the body. Cultures of fetal ovary, eight months, removed eight hours after death, showed a growth of the germinal epithelium. Granular cells were found in cultures of ovarian tissue removed from a woman who had cancer of the uterus.

**Menstruation and Tuberculosis.**—Maendl states that auscultation during menstruation reveals dry râles in the apices of tuberculous women, in whom at other times such signs are lacking. He regards this phenomenon as of help in diagnosis. A recent observation of Bricker also seems worth mentioning. He found that normal rabbits, inoculated with tubercle bacilli. began to lose weight at once, while castrated rabbits did not change for a long time. He believes that the removal of the ovaries produces changes which increase the body resistance against the tubercle bacilli.

**Menstrual Disturbances in the Feebleminded.**—Swanberg and Haynes report the study of 700 feebleminded women from this standpoint. In 425 menstruation was normal, in 177 there was a physiologic amenorrhea, and in 108 some form of pathologic menstrual disturbance was noted. The most common disorders were irregularity, amenorrhea, and dysmenorrhea. The percentage of menstrual disorders was in proportion to the degree of mental deficiency; the lower the mental state, the greater the number of pathologic cases. Amenorrhea and possibly oligomenorrhea were far more frequent among the lower types, imbeciles and idiots, while the vast majority of cases of dysmenorrhea were among the higher class, the morons.

**Menstruation and Hodgkin's Disease.**—Of 57 cases collected from the literature by Gemmell, all occurring in females, 39 were in women during menstrual life. In only 17 was the menstrual history available. In three menstruation was normal, in the other 14 there were varying degrees of oligomenorrhea, as far as complete amenorrhea in some cases. He suggests the use of ovarian extract in these cases, in addition to the usual treatment of the disease.

**Menstrual Peritonitis.**—A case of supposed "menstrual peritonitis" is reported by Adami. The patient was a girl of 14, who died on the third or fourth day of menstruation. Twelve hours after the completion of an athletic contest, the girl was seized with acute abdominal discomfort, then intense pain, followed by coma and death twelve hours after the onset. The autopsy showed the usual changes of menstruation, with a definite accumulation of translucent fluid in the pelvis. The examination of the abdominal fluid showed a pure culture of streptococcus in long chains. Adami suggests that during menstruation the mouth of the uterus is open, and that a negative pressure, such as might occur with various forms of exercise, might cause a sucking into the peritoneal cavity of some of the vaginal contents. Needless to say, such an explanation is purely speculative, and, furthermore, it lacks the ring of plausibility.

**Ovarian Therapy.**—PRESENT STATUS.—The author's present views on this subject were epitomized in a recent brief paper published under the auspices of the Council on Pharmacy and Chemistry of the American Medical Association, and it may therefore be justifiable to quote this paper in full:

The known facts as to the function of the ovary are sufficient to supply a rational basis for ovarian therapy. Especially important in this connection is the study of the phenomena produced by complete removal of ovarian tissue—the cessation of menstruation, the frequent appearance of troublesome subjective symptoms similar to those of the natural menopause, the occurrence of certain metabolic changes, etc. The obvious suggestion derived from such observations is that clinical symptoms thought to be due to ovarian deficiency might be cured or relieved by administering some form of ovarian substance. This fundamental idea has been subjected to some refinement as a result of studies aiming to stress some one or other of the ovarian constituents as the source of the active principle. Based on such investigations, several forms of ovarian therapy have developed—the administration of whole ovary substance, of corpus luteum extract alone, of the so-called ovarian residue, etc.

The first serious attempts at ovarian therapy were made in 1896 at the Landau clinic in Berlin, the preparation used being the fresh ovarian substance obtained from the cow or sow. Fraenkel, the foster father of the corpus luteum theory of menstruation, is also responsible for the use of the corpus luteum extract, which he employed in a small series of cases. The paper of Burnam in 1904 did much to popularize this form of therapy. A third preparation was suggested by Graves in 1919. It is obtained from that portion of the ovary remaining after removal of the corpus luteum. The study of the pharmacodynamics of the various forms of ovarian extract has until recent years yielded unimpressive results as regards the generative system. The most important fact gleaned has been that, in general, watery extracts are comparatively inert, and that the activity of the ovarian principle is in some way bound up with the lipoid content of the ovary. This point has a practical bearing in that it is a strong argument against the degreasing which is so often a step in the process of preparation of the commercial extracts.

The commercial extracts available are extracts of the whole ovary, corpus luteum extracts, and the ovarian residue. All these are procurable in the form of tablets, capsules, powder, or watery solutions (in ampules). The last named are probably inert, if the observations above quoted are correct. And yet they have achieved an enormous vogue. Of the other forms, it is difficult to outline indications for preference of whole ovary over corpus luteum, or vice versa. If any rule is possible, it would perhaps be that whole ovary is the more rational in developmental disorders of ovarian origin, whole corpus luteum extract is perhaps more desirable in those disturbances revolving about the menstrual function. The theory for the employment of ovarian residue is not convincing, and its use is not by any means as general as that of the other two. The watery extracts so widely used for hypodermic administration are probably inert, according to the best exidence available. Any good results obtained from their use are probably due either to the psychic factor or to the presence of protein factors which stimulate glandular structures generally, in accordance with the modern theory of protein therapy.

INDICATIONS.—*Functional Amenorrhea, Especially in Association with Adiposogenital Dystrophy.*—Here the indications are theoretically good, but the results are not very striking, even when combined with thyroid or pituitary extracts, as is usually done. And yet ovarian therapy is here more rational and much safer than the various so-called emmenogogue drugs; such as manganese or the vegetable oils. Ovarian therapy should not be used until the physician is satisfied that the amenorrhea is not, as is so often the case, a mere symptom of incipient tuberculosis, anemia, or other systemic disease.

*Menopausal Vasomotor Symptoms.*—Authors are almost unanimous in ascribing some virtue to ovarian therapy for this indication. Corpus luteum extracts are used perhaps more generally than those of the whole ovary. They appear to give some relief from the hot flushes, the heat flushes, the vertigo, and headache of the menopause. Often, on the other hand, they fail to help. There is some risk in drawing conclusions where one is dealing with such purely subjective symptoms, but the evidence of therapeutic value is greater with this than with any of the other indications for ovarian therapy.

*Uterine Hemorrhage.*—While a few writers report good results from ovarian therapy in certain forms of hemorrhage (especially the so-called functional hemorrhage of the menopause), this form of medication cannot be looked upon as offering very much hope of success—certainly no more than that offered by treatment with thyroid or posterior pituitary extracts. It should not be employed until after the diagnostic elimination of organic pelvic disease, especially cancer.

*Dysmenorrhea and Genital Hypoplasia* (Infantilism, etc.).—The only type of dysmenorrhea in which, even theoretically, organotherapy would seem to be indicated, is the so-called primary dysmenorrhea. This is commonly associated with varying degrees of underdevelopment of the uterus. This uterine hypoplasia is almost surely due to an endocrine defect of some form, although its exact nature is not known. Deficiency of the ovarian secretion is believed by many to be a factor, either primary or secondary, in this syndrome, and hence it is often used for its correction. Here again there is an obvious element of empiricism and hence it is not surprising that the results are anything but impressive.

*Sterility.*—What has been said of dysmenorrhea may be said of sterility. When combined with developmental deficiency of the uterus, organotherapy is a rational method of treatment. A few reports of good results are to be found in the literature (Fallenberg, Solomons), but far more frequently the results are disappointing. The essential importance of excluding the more common causes of sterility (inflammatory or other obstructions in one part or another of the genital tract, the male factor, etc.) need scarcely be emphasized.

*Obesity of Hypogenital Origin.*—This symptom is most often noted at the menopause, either natural or surgical. Certainly the administration of ovarian extracts for this indication is based on good grounds, and yet the results are not very striking, unless these extracts are combined with thyroid, in which case the latter is undoubtedly the potent agent.

*Vomiting of Pregnancy.*—This indication would not be entitled to the dignity of separate mention except that the hypodermic employment of corpus luteum extract for this symptom has achieved considerable vogue because of the recent publications of Hirst. The reasons given by this author for the form of treatment are speculative and illogical. When the method has been properly controlled, as in the study of King at the New Orleans Clinic, the results claimed by Hirst have not been confirmed. Moreover it is probable, as already stated, that the watery solutions used for hypodermic medication are inert. This method of treatment is a good illustration of organotherapy of the less desirable sort.

*Other Indications.*—One need only mention a list of indications for which ovarian therapy has been employed by various enthusiasts, usually without reason and almost always without result, *viz.*, repeated abortions, uterine fibroids, Graves' disease, deficient mammary secretion, epilepsy, pruritus vulvæ, etc. It may safely be said that no patient suffering from any of the above disorders will suffer from the omission of ovarian organotherapy.

In conclusion, it may again be emphasized that, rational as ovarian therapy appears to be in some conditions, the results are rarely striking and often nil to the level-headed observer. It cannot be assumed that a commercial extract can replace the normal secretion in the patient's body, or, for that matter, that it originally contains any of the active hormones of the ovary. Here lies the crux of the whole problem, whose solution will depend in large measure upon the work of the biochemist. Until this day, the physician who uses ovarian therapy should keep his feet on the ground, and not let himself be carried away by the exaggerated claims of those who have something to sell, or the ill-advised and premature reports of honest but deluded professional colleagues who have not yet learned the dangers lurking in the "post hoc propter hoc" method of reasoning. As I once heard a wise man say, "Ought we to assume, if the administration of cascara relieves constipation, that the constipated individual had been a victim of hypocascarism?" There can be little question as to the future importance of ovarian therapy; as regards its present importance, there is considerable room for discussion.

**Radium Therapy of Benign Uterine Bleeding.**—The treatment of bleeding associated with uterine cancer is of course subordinated to the treatment of the cancer itself, and this is a subject which we need scarcely consider in this chapter. It is with the benign hemorrhages that we are more directly concerned, especially those due to uterine myomata and those of so-called functional nature. In the latter, as we have already seen, the mucosa in a very large proportion of cases shows the condition designated as hyperplasia of the endometrium. Clark and Keene, from their study of 527 cases of these two groups, have drawn conclusions which may be taken as reflecting the opinions of those best qualified to speak on this subject. Radium and surgery must supplement each other in the treatment of cases of this type.

In the treatment of the hemorrhages of adolescent girls and young women, which resist less active measures, they advise caution in the use of radium. Only a very small initial dosage is employed. They suggest 50

Gms. for from three to four hours. The treatment is not to be repeated in less than six months, at which time it may be extended to from four to six hours. They have had no failures following the second application, although cases of this group have been very infrequent.

The functional bleeding of the menopause furnishes perhaps the clearest and most satisfactory indication for radiotherapy. The importance of excluding malignancy, usually by diagnostic curettage, is obvious. As Clark and Keene state, radiotherapy in these cases "is effective, it is quick in giving relief, the treatment does not incapacitate the patient, it is safe, and it is followed by practically no immediate disabling sequelæ or remote ill effects."

With regard to the treatment of hemorrhage during active reproductive life, great care is necessary in the employment of radiation, chiefly because of the risk of sterilizing the patient. There are many radiologists who believe that this risk can be almost entirely obviated by using small dosage, but it is probable that most gynecologists will continue to use this form of therapy for this group of cases only where all other measures fail. Certainly the patient is entitled to the confidence of the surgeon when radiotherapy is contemplated, and her own preference, after a fair presentation of the case, will often be a satisfying guide to the surgeon in his management of the case.

With regard to the bleeding so often seen with uterine myomata, opinion has crystallized fairly well. Where hemorrhage is the chief symptom of such tumors, and where they do not exceed the size of a three (some say four) months' pregnancy, radiotherapy is indicated. When they are larger than the size above indicated, when they are complicated by pelvic inflammatory disease, and when they are causing serious pressure symptoms, radiotherapy is contraindicated. Calcified and large submucous tumors are also considered by Clark and Keene as unsuitable for irradiation. Finally, it need scarcely be said that the treatment of myomata occurring in young women is subject to the same restrictions, based on the danger of sterilization, which have been mentioned above in connection with the subject of functional hemorrhage.

Graves calls attention to certain unpleasant symptoms which may be noted after the use of radium in cases of uterine hemorrhage. He mentions especially nausea, continuance or reappearance of the bleeding, leukorrhea, pain, acute nephritis, and nervous symptoms.

## LITERATURE

1. Stockard and Papanicalou. The Existence of a Typical Œstrous Cycle in the Guinea-Pig, with a Study of Its Histological and Physiological Changes. Am. J. Anat., 1917, 22, 225.
2. Allen, Doisy, *et al.* The Hormon of the Ovarian Follicle; Its Localization and Action in Test Animals, etc. Am. J. Anat., 1924, 34, 133.
3. Allen and Doisy. The Induction of a Sexually Mature Condition in

Immature Females by Injection of the Ovarian Follicular Hormone. Am. J. Physiol., 1924, 69, 577.
4. Novak and TeLinde. The Endometrium of the Menstruating Uterus. J. Am. M. Ass., 1924, 83, 900.
5. Schick. Das Menstruationsgift. Wien. klin. Wchnschr., 1920, 19, 1.
6. Macht and Lubin. Phyto-pharmacologic Study of Menstrual Toxin. J. Pharmacol. & Exper. Therap., 1924, 22, 413.
7. Labhardt. Zur Frage des Menstruationsgiftes. Zentralbl. f. Gynäk., 1924, 48, 2626.
8. Wakeman. Basal Metabolism and Menstrual Cycle. J. Biol. Chem., 1923, 56, 555.
9. Heilig. Menstruationsstudien-Zuckerstoffwechsel. Wien. klin. Wchnschr., 1924, 3, 576.
10. Bond. "Ammonia Coefficient" in Menstruation. Lancet, 1922, 2, 957.
11. Amos. Variations of Blood Pressure During Menstruation. Lancet, 1922, 2, 956.
12. Council on Pharmacy and Chemistry of the American Medical Association. Report on Benzyl Compounds. J. Am. M. Ass., 1924, 83, 1864.
13. Gruber and Shackelford. Pharmacology of Benzyl Alcohol and Its Esters. J. Lab. & Clin. Med., 1924, 9, 685.
14. Novak and Martzloff. Hyperplasia of the Endometrium. Am. J. Obst. & Gynec., 1924, 8, 385.
15. Sampson. The Influence of Ectopic Pregnancy on the Uterus, etc. Tr. Am. Gynec. Soc., 1913, 38, 121.
16. Polak and Wolfe. A Further Study of the Origin of Uterine Bleeding in Ectopic Pregnancy. Am. J. Obst. & Gynec., 1924, 8, 730.
17. Novak and Darner. The Correlation of Uterine and Tubal Changes in Tubal Gestation. Am. J. Obst. & Gynec., 1925, 9, 295.
18. Stickel and Zondek. Klinische Untersuchungen Ueber den Wert der Organotherapie bei Ovarielles Blutungen. Ztschr. f. Geburtsh. u. Gynäk., 1923, 85, 83.
19. Hornung. Das Verhalten der Thrombocyten und ihre Beinflussung durch Kalkmedikation. Zentralbl. f. Gynäk., 1923, 47, 1285.
20. Roth. Ueber vikariiende Menstruation. Monatschr. f. Geburtsh. u. Gynæk., 1920, 51, 41.
21. Tuffier. Transposition of the Ovary with Its Vascular Pedicle into the Uterus After Salpingectomy. Surg. Gynec. & Obst., 1924, 39, 401.
22. Bell. Nature of Ovarian Function. Lancet, 1920, 2, 879.
23. Sippel. Die Ovarientransplantation bei herabgesetzter und fehlender Genitalfunktion. Arch. f. Gynæk., 1923, 118, 445.
24. Martin. Ovarian Transplantation. Surg., Gynec. & Obst., 1922, 35, 573.
25. Zondek and Wolff. Zur Züchtung von menschlichem ovarial Gewebe in vitro. Zentralbl. f. Gynäk., 1924, 48, 2193.
26. Maendl. Ueber die Verwertung der Mensesreaktion zur Beurtheilung der Aktivität tuberkulöser Krankheitserscheinungen insbesondere der Lungen. Wien. klin. Wchnschr., 1924, 37, 440.
27. Swanberg and Haynes. Menstrual Disturbances in the Feebleminded. J. Ment. & Nerv. Dis., 1919, 50, 224.

28. GEMMELL. Menstruation and Pregnancy in Lymphadenoma (Hodgkin's Disease). J. Obst. & Gynæc. Brit. Emp., 1923, 30, 373.
29. ADAMI. Fulminant Menstrual Peritonitis. J. Obst. & Gynæc. Brit. Emp., 1922, 29, 104.
30. NOVAK. Ovarian Therapy. J. Am. M. Ass., 1924, 83, 2017.
31. CLARK AND KEENE. Uterine Hemorrhage of Benign Origin Treated by Irradiation. J. Am. M. Ass., 1922, 79, 546.
32. GRAVES. Radium Treatment of Non-Malignant Uterine Bleeding. N. York M. J., 1920, 111, 969.

# EXTRA-UTERINE PREGNANCY

EDWARD A. SCHUMANN, M.D.

## APPENDIX

During the past four years there has accumulated a fairly large literature concerning ectopic pregnancy, but no very radical views as to its pathology, symptomatology, or treatment have gained acceptance. The most important progress has resulted from the widespread attempt to improve the treatment of abdominal pregnancy, with special reference to the management of the ectopic placenta. This work will be discussed in detail below. Some new diagnostic symptoms and signs have been elicited, the pathology of the condition has undergone careful scrutiny but in general the principles laid down in the body of this book remain unchanged.

A brief review of the more important contributions since 1921 follows.

**Etiology of Extra-Uterine Pregnancy.**—The generally accepted cause of tubal pregnancy, obstruction of the tubal canal from within its lumen, carries with it the query as to whether such obstruction is more generally postinflammatory in origin or whether there are present congenital malformation of the tubes. Schoenholz (*Arch. f. Gynæk.* 1923. 120:44) made anatomic examination of 32 pregnant tubes and in 26 cases he found a mesh or diverticulum formation which he considers as paramount in etiology. This observer holds that the mesh formation is not comparable to the changes in the tubal mucosa brought about by inflammatory change and considers the process a congenital anomaly.

Studies of large numbers of tubes at the seat of gestation, conclusively prove, however, that no one cause may be assigned for the production of these lesions. Peritoneal adhesions causing stenosis by occlusion from without, the tubal mucosa presenting no abnormalities whatever, with an ovum implanted distal to the obstruction form too common a clinical picture to be ignored. So, also, the observation of plastic exudate gluing together folds of the mucosa, together with the evidences of a healing salpingitis are very usual findings, while congenital anomalies and diverticula are somewhat uncommon.

**Cause of Uterine Bleeding in Ectopic Pregnancy.**—Polak and Welton (Polak, John O., and Welton, T. S. *Am. J. Obst. & Gynec.* 1922.

3:164) have shown that uterine bleeding does not occur while a tubal ovum is healthy and development is proceeding. When there is ovular unrest, however, some damage being done to the tubal embryo by interovular hemorrhage and hemorrhage into its sac, there is bleeding from the uterine decidua (which is always found in greater or less degree in cases of tubal pregnancy), as well as from the decidual areas in the tube.

While tubal pregnancy is being terminated the tube undergoes some wavelike intermittent contractions, which are transmitted to the uterus when this organ in turn contracts as in abortion, giving rise to bleeding and separation of its decidua. In addition, should the tubal gestation be situated near the uterine end of the tube, there is usually some blood forced into the uterine cavity from the tube itself.

The uterine bleeding, which is usually small in amount, may continue for a considerable time after the attack of abdominal pain which apparently marks the destruction of the embryo. This is due to the fact that the termination of the tubal pregnancy is not necessarily at once complete, chorionic villi remaining alive, exerting their stimulus upon the uterus (Polak and Welton).

**Termination of Tubal Pregnancy.**—Recent literature contains several important contributions to this subject, the trend of thought being rather to discredit the long held view that tubal abortion is one of the two usual end-results of tubal implantation of the ovum. Litzenberg (Litzenberg. J. C. *Tr. Amer. Gynec. Soc.* 1920. 239), describes the microscopic anatomy in a series of cases where the pregnant tube was cut parallel to its long axis, serial section of the whole tube being so studied. He maintains that the condition called tubal abortion is not, strictly speaking, an abortion, analogous to a uterine abortion, *i.e.*, a separation of the ovum from its attachment and extrusion by the activity of the musculature of the tubes. If the implantation is near the ostium abdominale it may grow out from the fimbriated extremity by simply increasing in size, protruding from the end of the tube but not detached from its imbedding in the tubal wall.

If the implantation is near the uterine end of the tube the termination may be by internal rupture through the inner ovum capsule into the tube lumen, or, rarely, separation of the ovum, in which case it perishes, may become a tubal mole, or it may be pushed along toward the fimbriated end by the hemorrhage, but not by the tube muscle.

McDonald has advanced the theory that tubal pregnancy really takes place outside the tubal mucosal canal and between the muscular coats of the tube wall. With the growth of the ovum there is dissection of the muscular coats of the tube and destruction of the tissue by the invading trophoblast.

The first common accident is intramural extravasation of blood which precedes the first symptom of tubal pregnancy. Fimbrial rupture follows in two-thirds of the cases. Fimbrial rupture often occurs through dissection of the muscular coats to their juncture with the mucosa at the fimbrial and hemorrhagic discharge at the end of the tube through a break in the tissue (McDonald, Ellice. *Am. J. Obst. & Gynec.* 1923. 6:73).

These opinions are not valid, in the judgment of the writer, since the mechanisms described by Litzenberg in the development of what he terms internal rupture is precisely that of incomplete uterine abortion; death and extrusion of the embryo with hemorrhage and the continued attachment of the sac of the ovum to the uterine wall, until its separation is accomplished by a sort of sloughing or, indeed, by manual measures. So far as McDonald's fimbrial rupture is concerned, this accident probably does occur, but it certainly does not constitute a usual termination, since the protrusion of the ovum directly through the fimbriated extremity of the tubes has been demonstrated in so large a series of cases.

A most remarkable termination is that reported by Streeter (Streeter, George L. *J. Am. M. Ass.* 1923. 80:989):

"The author believes this is the first reported case in which a human ovum became implanted and underwent development entirely outside the abdominal cavity. A woman, aged 25, had been married four years. She had had one abortion but no children. When first seen she exhibited a mass the size of a cherry in the lower abdominal region at the upper end of a scar from a previous operation. A provisional diagnosis of wound-hernia was made. When seen two weeks later the swelling had doubled in size, and on account of its rapid growth an exploratory examination was decided on, the swelling at this time having reached the size of a hen's egg. Operation disclosed, just beneath the skin, embedded in the superficial fascia, a relatively thin-walled and partially transparent cyst, which on removal proved to be an intact chorionic sac, and on being opened was found to contain a well formed embryo. The operative area was carefully examined, but no opening through the deep fascia or connection with the abdomen could be found. Nor was there any enveloping capsule or any structure other than is normally present in the abdominal fascia, although there seemed to be some enlargement of the blood-vessels leading to the area of implantation. It appeared that two years before the patient had had a ventral fixation of the uterus and the surgeon had adopted that procedure in which the round ligaments are pulled through the rectus muscles. It is possible that he mistook the fallopian tube for the round ligament or drew the tube through the rectus muscle along with the round ligament. It is assumed that the fertilized ovum in this case was arrested at the tubal kink and, eroding through the mucosa of the tube wall, continued its development in the loose tissues superficial to the rectus muscle."

A detailed study of the specimen showed that the chorion and its contained embryo appeared to have grown about as well as they would have had the implantation occurred in the uterine mucosa. In general form and microscopic structure they could not be distinguished from normally implanted ova of the same stage of development. The tissues of the embryo showed beginning degenerative changes indicating that it had reached its maximum development and that the heart had stopped before the time of operation. The relative development of the hands, feet, ears, eyes, and mouth region was normal for the length of the embryo, and corresponded to about the end of the eighth week. The external genitalia were developed in proportion to the other parts of the body and were female in type. Whereas the embryo showed a development of eight weeks, the clinical record obtained from the patient gave a menstrual age of ten weeks, the discrepancy being accounted for by the retardation and arrest in development.

**Multiple Tubal Pregnancy.**—*Tubal Twinning.*—It has been shown that the relative frequency of single ovum twins as compared to the double ovum variety is far greater in tubal than in uterine pregnancy and a valid and lucid explanation of this phenomenon is suggested by Arey (Arey, Leslie B. *Am. J. Obst. & Gynec.* 1923. 5:163), who is hereafter quoted *in extenso.*

It seems to be definitely proved (by the experiments of Stockard and others) that the primary cause of an abnormal development including twins is a developmental inhibition or arrest; the exact type of deformity that results depends solely on the precise moment when the interruption occurs. The direct application to twinning is as follows: The periphery of the blastoderm possesses many points where an embryonic axis might arise. In ordinary single development one such growing point, apparently by virtue of its favorable positional advantage, gives the supremacy and suppresses all other potential points, just as the terminal bud does the lateral ones in some plants.

If, however, the developmental rate is slowed at the critical moment when this axis is about to assert its dominance, its advantage is then lost and one or more neighboring points can now compete on more equal terms and may assert themselves as additional embryonic axes. If these growing points are far apart separate individuals result; if nearer together, various degrees of conjoining. The critical moment for twinning is at the onset of gastrulation which in mammals corresponds to the formation of a primitive streak. Thus the production of twins (separate or conjoined) and all non-hereditary malformations of organs and parts, are reducible to a single causative factor, namely, a properly timed developmental onset.

The application of the principle to the ovum in extra-uterine pregnancy lies in the fact that the ovum is subject to delay before implantation due to the impediments to its passage through the tube until it reaches such size that it can no longer reach the uterine cavity, or the ovum may be incarcerated in diverticula or blind passages where it must perforce remain.

FIG. 1.—PHOTOGRAPH OF 12.3 MILLIMETER HUMAN TUBAL TWIN EMBRYOS ATTACHED TO A COMMON YOLK SAC. × 2.3.

FIGS. 2 and 3.—ADDITIONAL PHOTOGRAPHS OF THE COMMON YOLK SAC SHOWN IN FIGURE 1. The origin of the separate yolk stalks is apparent. × 2.3.

FIG. 4.—PHOTOGRAPH OF A PREGNANT HUMAN UTERINE TUBE. Part of the wall has been removed to show the twin embryos in place. The single yolk sac belongs to the 11.5 millimeter embryo at the left. The 12.0 millimeter embryo at the right lacks both yolk sac and stalk. × 1.7.

FIG. 5.—PHOTOMICROGRAPH OF A SECTION THROUGH THE UMBILICAL CORD OF THE EMBRYO AT THE LEFT IN FIGURE 4. The yolk stalk lies in a cœlomic extension. The level is too far distad to include the allantois. × 24.

FIG. 6.—PHOTOMICROGRAPH OF A SECTION THROUGH THE UMBILICAL CORD OF THE EMBRYO AT THE RIGHT IN FIGURE 4. There is no trace of a yolk stalk. The delicate tube below is the allantois. × 24.

The implantation of the ovum has therefore been greatly delayed, and furthermore its imbedding in the tubal mucosa is always associated with a deficiency or oxygenation of the growing embryo and a consequent developmental arrest at the critical moment for twinning. Two embryonic axes are apt to result with the production of monochorial twins. Checks, permanent or temporary, while the chorion is struggling to overcome natural deficiencies in its nidus are sufficient to account for excessive twinning and the frequency of double malformations in extra-uterine fetus.

In another valuable contribution Arey (Arey, L. B. *Surg., Gynec. & Obst.* 1923. 36:407), collected the reported cases of tubal twins and those of plural pregnancies, where one fetus occupied the tube, the other being implanted in its normal nidus, the uterine cavity.

Arey presents 40 authentic cases, which withstand critical analysis, 8 presumptive ones, and 4 which are possible but doubtful.

**Superfetation and Superfecundation in Tubal Pregnancy.**—Discussion of multiple tubal pregnancy leads naturally to a consideration of the vexed question of superfetation in these cases. The generally

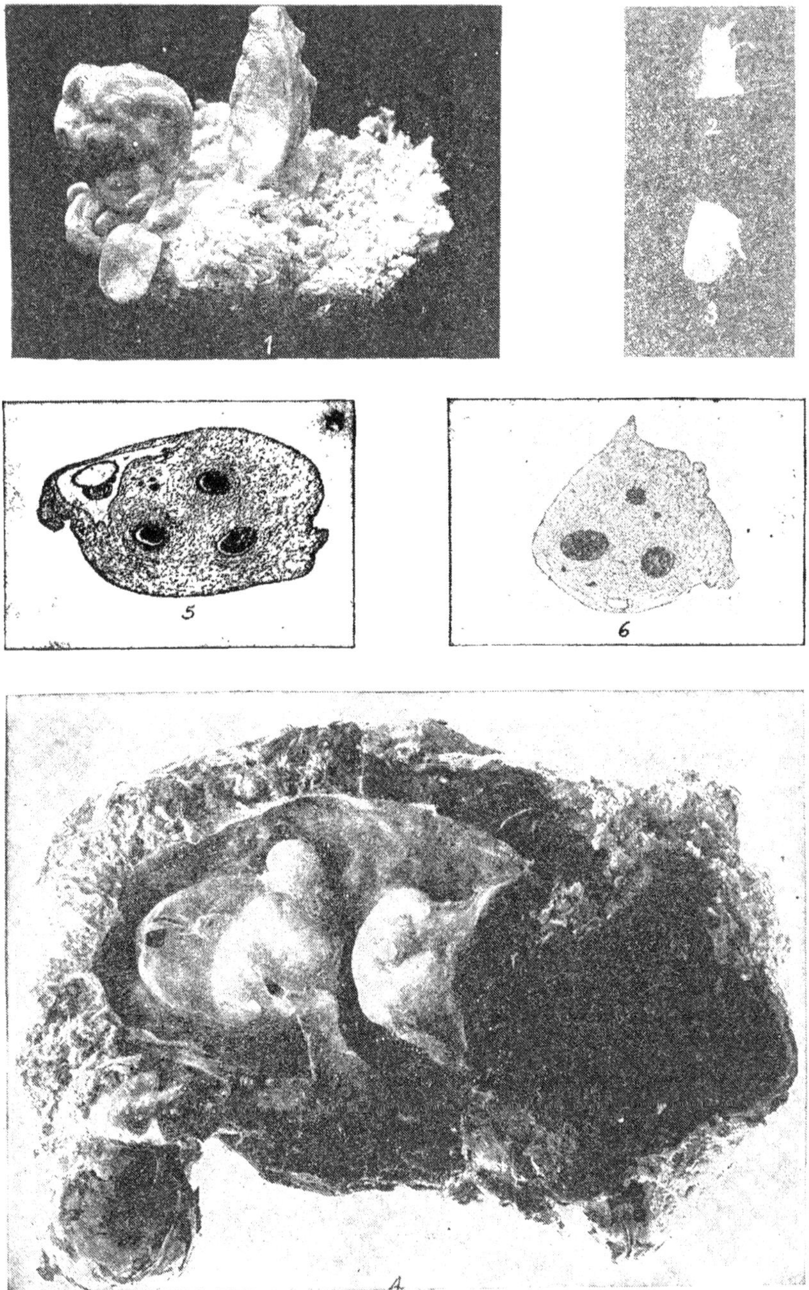


From Arey, *Surg., Gyn. & Obst.*, Mar. 1923.

FOR LEGENDS, SEE OPPOSITE PAGE.

accepted definition of superfecundation as well stated by Radasch (Radasch, H. E. *Surg., Gynec. & Obst.* 1921. 32:339), is that condition in which two or more ova belonging to or originating at the same ovulation period are fertilized from sperm from coitus practiced at different times by the same or another male. The ova may originate from one or both ovaries, but in the latter case the ovulation must be practically simultaneous.

Superfetation is the fertilization of two or more ova that belong to or originate at different ovular periods by sperm from coitus at the same or different times by the same or another male. This assumes a pregnancy superimposed upon another by the fertilization of an ovum of a later date.

The essential difference between the two terms lies in the fact that in the former instance the ova are separately fertilized but themselves are of the same maturity, that is they are products of the same ovulation period, while in the latter, the ova are of different ages, products of two ovulation periods. The possibility of the occurrence of these phenomena is still in doubt, the Germans usually denying its existence while the French and American observers credit it.

Reported cases are few, De Lee recording one specimen shown at the Chicago Gynecological Society where two extra-uterine pregnancies of different dates had been removed at operation.

**Abdominal Pregnancy.**—The recent literature contains constantly increasing numbers of case reports dealing with this interesting condition. From the very nature of the lesson, bizarre and dramatic findings are to be expected and the anticipation of such phenomena is not infrequently exceeded by the exposure of the lesson present. Reported cases of abdominal pregnancy should always include a detailed account of the location and attachment of the placenta and the method of dealing with it since this phase of the subject is not completely settled yet and requires the cumulative experience of many obstetricians to determine the optimum procedure.

The tendency is steadily growing to regard the placenta as a digestible, autogenous tissue mass and to leave it undisturbed, the child and membranes as well as any pathological pelvic organs being removed and the abdomen closed without drainage.

Many clinical observations seem to substantiate the view that this way of handling the placenta offers the lowest mortality yet achieved and immeasurably reduces the maternal morbidity since the older plans of marsupialization with slow necrosis and sloughing of the placenta predicates many weeks of hospitalization and a high incidence of terminal defect of the abdominal parietes, subsequent operation being necessary to repair the herniæ.

In Jewett's case (Jewett, Wm. A. *Am. J. Obst. & Gynec.* 1923. 5:176), the placenta was very large and was firmly attached to the right side of the posterior surface of the uterus, the right broad ligament extending into the culdesac and up on the posterior pelvic wall as far as the brim of the pelvis overlying the iliac vessels of that side. As it was evident that removal must be attended by serious hemorrhage, the placenta was left in situ, the cord ligated and cut close to its insertion. The patient made an uneventful recovery and left the hospital in two weeks. Pelvic examination at frequent intervals showed a gradual decrease in the size of the placenta, during the first six months after the operation, but no apparent diminution during the next six months. It is, however, more movable in the pelvis and much less sensitive. The patient appears to be perfectly well.

While it is not yet time to lay down a definite rule, it would seem that in uninfected patients, the abdominally situated ectopic placenta will undergo at least partial absorption and that it is not a source of great danger to the patient if left in situ and the abdomen closed. On the other hand, attempts at its removal are often fraught with such grave danger from hemorrhage while the old plan of marsupialization, stitching the peritoneum around the placenta and packing the cavity with gauze, carries with it such certainty of prolonged convalescence, infection of the sloughing mass and probability of a permanent damage to the integrity of the abdominal wall, that almost any plan of treatment would seem preferable. The leaving of the placenta, with, possibly, a second operation to remove the unabsorbed remainder, after some months have elapsed, seems to offer the best solution as yet devised.

*Two Abdominal Pregnancies in the Same Patient, Following Supravaginal Hysterectomy.*—McMillan (McMillan, W. A. *West Va. M. J.* 1921. 16:183) reports a case in which a supravaginal hysterectomy was performed for infection in a patient 18 years of age. The right ovary and about 1½ inches of the distal end of the right tube were left in. Eighteen months later abdominal pregnancy was diagnosed and upon section a recently dead infant of 8½ pounds weight was found enveloped in its ruptured amniotic sac. The placenta was situated in the left flank under the spleen and was slowly separated. Twelve months later this patient reported with a second pregnancy which proceeded until the seventh month, when a four-pound dead infant was removed by section. Hemorrhage resulted in the death of the mother.

**Diagnosis of Tubal Pregnancy.**—New Diagnostic Signs.—*Sud-*

*den Acute Pain in the Shoulder, Indicating Subphrenic Blood Extravasation.*—Rubin (Rubin, I. C. *J. Am. M. Ass.*, 1923. 80:1050) states that the shoulder pains so commonly noted as accompanying artificial subphrenic pneumoperitoneum are comparable to those due to the sudden accumulation of fluid in the subphrenic space. The pain produced in the diaphragmatic area is referred to the shoulders by sensitized cutaneous nerves of the cervical segments, the phrenic nerve having its origin in the third, fourth, and fifth cervical cord segments and connecting with cervical peripheral nerves supplying the shoulder girdle.

In ruptured ectopic pregnancies with extensive hemoperitoneum, bilateral shoulder pains are present but affect more intensely the shoulder corresponding to the side of the tubal rupture.

When the hemorrhage is not extensive and is confined to one side, the shoulder pain will indicate the side of the rupture. This sign should be extremely valuable if continued observation corroborates the findings. In the experience of the writer patients with massive hemorrhage are usually very ill and in shock and despite careful history taking he has been unable to elicit this symptom except in very scattered instances. When the hemorrhage was small he was only once able to get a report of shoulder pain from a patient.

*Bluish Discoloration about the Umbilicus; Cullen's Sign.*—This interesting phenomenon to which attention has been directed elsewhere in this book, is being occasionally noted, but with no degree of uniformity.

In an analysis of 50 cases of ectopic pregnancy operated upon recently at Johns Hopkins Hospital, Brady found no evidence of this sign (Brady, Leo. *Johns Hopkins Hospital Bull.* 1923. 34:152). The author has reported a case wherein the bluish discoloration about the umbilicus was very marked, and was regarded as corroborative of the diagnosis of ectopic pregnancy which was based upon a highly suggestive symptom complex. At operation there was found a normal intra-uterine pregnancy and bilateral acute purulent salpingitis, there being no blood present in the abdominal cavity at all (Schumann, E. A. *Am. J. Obst. & Gynec.* 1923. 6:632). In view of these findings, it follows that while an interesting and suggestive observation periumbilical ecchymosis is not in any sense pathognomonic of abdominal hemorrhage nor does its absence weaken such diagnosis in any given case.

**Chemical Tests for Ectopic Pregnancy.**—Phlorizin glycosuria has been used to some extent as a test for pregnancy, glycosuria appearing in most pregnant women a half hour after the injection; in the first half of pregnancy the reaction is more readily positive than in the second half. Paruzza finds this test a most valuable one in determining the existence of extra-uterine pregnancy (Paruzza, Mario P. *Riv. di Ostet. e ginec. prat.* Palermo, 1924, 6:76).

In doubtful cases the positive phlorizin reaction may contribute to point the way to an exact evaluation of the syndrome of ectopic gestation. Paruzza cites four cases in which this test was strongly positive while the ovum was still uninjured or immediately after rupture but became negative in the presence of hematoceles attending the definite termination of an extra-uterine pregnancy.

These observations are extremely important and should be verified and their degree of accuracy determined upon.

TREATMENT.—No radical change in the treatment of ectopic pregnancy has been offered although the trend against deferred operation seems to be steadily growing, the majority of these reporting series of cases advocating immediate operation in all cases.

The propriety of removing the affected tube or, if possible, of conserving it, removing the ovum and resecting the diseased portion of the tube is still under discussion. Cases of normal pregnancies following salpingotomy are recorded, but in final analysis it appears that the danger of repeated tubal gestation so outweighs the probabilities of normal pregnancy in these cases that salpingectomy is the procedure of choice except when, the remaining tube being absent or hopelessly diseased, the patient elects to retain even the remote possibility of future childbearing.

*Reinfusion of Blood.*—The infusion of the free blood found in the peritoneal cavity in cases of ruptured ectopic pregnancy directly back into the blood stream has been performed in a number of instances, most operators describing their results as excellent. In a very complete paper Klopp (Klopp, E. J. *Tr. Am. Surg. Ass.* 1922. 40:203) reviews the subject, reporting 11 cases of his own. Thies of Leipzig appears to have first suggested this procedure (Thies, J., *Zentralbl. f. Gynäk.* 1914. 38:34:1191) of collecting the blood from a ruptured extra-uterine pregnancy with a spoon, straining it through double-ply muslin and diluting with salt solution in the proportion of 3 to 2. Thies's three patients recovered with uneventful convalescence.

Before applying the method the blood found in other cases free in the abdominal cavity had been examined and found sterile, and the erythrocytes were unimpaired.

This paper was followed by those of Lichtenstein, Armin, Topler, and many others. (For a complete survey of the literature see Klopp's paper quoted above.)

The technic according to Klopp is to bail the blood out of the abdominal cavity with a cup and transfer it to a graduate placed in a water bath. The cubital veins having been prepared a canula is inserted and after running a small quantity of salt solution into the vein through a funnel, the blood is strained through six-ply fine meshed gauze, directly into the funnel. Citration seems to be unnecessary. In Klopp cases the amount of blood reinfused varied from 300 to 900 c.c. This author concludes that reinfusion should not be used routinely in cases of ruptured ectopic pregnancy, but should be employed in the cases in which the loss of blood has caused desperate symptoms.

Zimmerman (Zimmerman, R. *Ztschr. f. Geburtsh. u. Gynäk.* 1921. 84:355) believes one should take advantage of the resorptive power of the peritoneum in cases of intra-abdominal hemorrhage.

In instances of non-infected intra-peritoneal blood effusion during tubal pregnancy it is advised that clots be removed, leaving the fluid blood intact. The latter is defibrinated and therefore no longer coagulates and is rapidly and completely resorbed, so that the majority of the erythrocytes reach the general circulation in a state of good functional ability. Intravenous transfusion of the effused blood should only be carried out when the condition of the patient becomes grave during the operative procedures.

In as much as reinfusion is considered as indicated only when the blood loss is great, it seems that the loss of time necessary to bail out any appreciable amount of blood from the abdomen will more than offset any advantage gained. Furthermore, since this blood is defibrinated and therefore has no further value in inducing coagulation, so necessary a factor where severe hemorrhage has taken place, the procedure is of but little value, in the opinion of the writer.

A very rapid operation, leaving as much of the free blood as may be in the abdomen for its future resorption, together with the prompt transfusion of fresh blood from a properly selected donor offers far greater probabilities of success.

In addition, while no instances of bacteriemia are recorded as following the reinfusion of blood, the necessary manipulation will certainly increase the danger of the contamination of the blood so utilized.

# CESAREAN SECTION

FRANKLIN S. NEWELL, M.D.

## APPENDIX

Since the publication of this monograph little or no change has taken place in our attitude toward cesarean section. A cursory study of the recent literature on the subject combined with an examination of the reports of the causes of death in the parturient state in various sections of the country from which the reports are available has strengthened our opinion that cesarean section is at the present time the most abused operation in obstetrics. Apparently from one-fourth to one-third of the deaths occurring during parturition follow cesarean section for different indications, and such investigations as we have been able to make in regard to the indications for the operation in the fatal cases point to the fact that cesarean section is resorted to in a large proportion of the cases on account of its ease of performance, in spite of the fact that definite contra-indications for the classical operation, at least, are present, and that the patients should have been delivered by other means.

**Analysis of Mortality.**—The majority of the fatal cases whose history we have been able to trace had been many hours in labor, often with ruptured membranes for twenty-four hours or longer, and in many instances cesarean section had been performed after a failure at attempts to deliver by forceps. A careful study of the indications and contra-indications in the given case and an intelligent application of the rules which have been formulated to govern the choice of operation in such cases would have resulted in many fewer cesarean sections and a corresponding diminution in the maternal mortality in cases which are unfit for abdominal surgery. More children would undoubtedly have been lost, but many mothers would have been saved.

As we have tried to make clear, our firm belief is that the only safe time for the conservative cesarean section is before labor begins or early in labor, and any neglect of this principle is sure to be attended by a high mortality. This presupposes a careful study of the patient and the selection of the method of delivery preferably before labor begins, and certainly early in labor. In general practice comparatively few patients are properly studied until labor has been in progress for some time, and as a rule the consultant who is called late in labor decides cesarean section is necessary to save the child and proceeds at once to the operation without any regard for the possibility of infection and death of the mother. The mortality in cesarean section will continue to be high until careful prenatal study, including pelvic mensuration and examination under anesthesia, becomes universal so that the operation is performed at the time of election instead of late in labor.

Another fruitful cause for the mortality in cesarean section is the fact that at the present time it is the most popular method of delivering patients with eclampsia. These patients are naturally poor risks for abdominal surgery, being thoroughly toxic in the first place, and seriously shocked by the occurrence of convulsions in the second place. Furthermore, most of them show suppression of urine to such a degree that no surgeon would consider them as proper risks for other surgical procedures. Cesarean section is probably the most fatal method employed to-day in the treatment of eclampsia, and yet in this country at least is the most popular method, and this in spite of the fact that it has been definitely proved that the conservative treatment of eclampsia, *i.e.,* the Stroganoff treatment, gives far better results than any surgical procedure.

We still believe that in clean cases with no question of uterine infection the classical operation is the most satisfactory procedure. When, however, any doubt exists as to uterine infection, as for instance in cases who have been long in labor, who have been subjected to repeated vaginal examinations, or who have had ruptured membranes for some time, and especially in those who have been subjected to attempted delivery by forceps, the classical cesarean section is attended by too high a mortality and morbidity to warrant its performance. In these cases an extraperitoneal cesarean section, as by the methods of Latsko and Küstner, or, even better, a transperitoneal suprasymphyseal operation by the method described by Beck gives better results. We do not believe in the substitution of extra- or transperitoneal operations for the classical operation in clean cases, but in the doubtful cases there is no question but the results are better. In our experience, however, the convalescence is not as smooth as the advocates of the operation would lead us to believe, but the main point is that though the convalescence may be stormy the mortality is reduced.

We do not believe that any conservative operation should be performed on patients who are considered definitely infected. In these cases, if cesarean section is absolutely necessary, the operation should be completed by the removal of the uterus either by supravaginal amputation or by a complete hysterectomy.

In our experience with the various extra- and transperitoneal operations several of which have been described in the text, the Beck operation would seem to be the most satisfactory method described at present. Since this operation has not been included among the operations previously described, a brief description follows.

**Beck Operation.**—The abdomen is opened in the midline by an incision extending from a point just below the umbilicus to the symphysis pubis. If the patient has been in labor for any considerable time the peritoneal attachment in the region of the bladder reflection will be found markedly loosened. The loose peritoneum just above the region of the bladder reflection is incised transversely. Early in labor there may be some difficulty in properly exposing this area but this will be overcome by placing the patient in a moderate Trendelenburg position. Late in labor the field of operation is easily exposed without resorting to the Trendelenburg posture. The bladder and peritoneum are dissected off the anterior surface of the uterus as in abdominal hysterectomy. The peritoneum on the upper side of the incision is then carefully dissected free from its attachment to the uterus. This is best done by passing a pair of scissors gently under the peritoneum in the line of cleavage. They are then opened and withdrawn, thus freeing the peritoneum from the underlying tissues. If this is done several times on each side, a good peritoneal flap is obtained. The two peritoneal flaps are then held back by retractors, and the lower segment of the uterus and upper portion of the cervix are exposed. Considerable hemorrhage may be met with at this point but it is readily controlled in most cases by pressure with gauze packs.

In as much as the patients on whom we do this operation are in the doubtful class as far as asepsis goes, it is well to wall off the abdominal cavity carefully to prevent contamination by the spill. This is accomplished by gauze packs aided by pressure with the hands of an assistant on either side of the uterus.

A small stab wound is made in the midline of the uterus and this is lengthened by means of a scissors, the incision being made first in the lowest portion of the wound and then extended upwards. There is no danger of injury to the bladder as it is held out of the way by means of a retractor. One hand is then passed into the uterine cavity, a finger inserted into the mouth of the child, and the face is rotated anteriorly and held in the wound. Forceps are then applied to the sides of the head and delivery is accomplished as in a face presentation. Before attempting to remove the placenta and membranes a deep traction suture is passed through the wall of the uterus just below the lower angle of the wound. This will facilitate closure of the wound since it will prevent retraction of the lower angle of the wound into the pelvis. A similar traction suture is placed just above the upper angle of the incision. Traction on these sutures by an assistant holds the wound in a proper position for suture and also helps to wall off the peritoneal cavity. The placenta and membranes are then manually removed or pushed through the cervix into the vagina. An ampule of pituitrin is injected directly into the wall of the uterus. The wound is closed by two series of interrupted chromic catgut sutures, the first passing through the uterine wall down to the endometrium. The suture should begin at the upper angle and end at the lower, special pains being taken to close each angle. The second series should include about half the thickness of the muscle wound, each suture being placed midway between the deeper ones. The traction sutures are then tied, thus bringing together any fibers which may have been torn beyond the line of incision. The sutures are then cut and a large portion of the wound drops into the pelvis.

The upper peritoneal flap is then brought down over the upper portion of the closed uterine incision and is fastened by several interrupted catgut sutures, avoiding the uterine suture in the midline. It is best that these sutures should not be passed into the uterine cavity. The bladder reflection is then carried one centimeter above the transverse incision, overlapping the upper peritoneal flap and thoroughly sealing the uterine wound, the flap being held in place by superficial catgut sutures.

In our experience with this operation the convalescence is not as smooth as has been commonly stated, most of the patients running a more or less elevated temperature for several days, but the principal point is that they eventually recover whereas if the classical operation is done under such circumstances a maternal mortality of at least 10 per cent is to be expected, and in addition a high morbidity.

We do not feel that this operation is adequate when the uterus is believed to be definitely infected and favor hysterectomy in such cases instead of leaving the septic uterus to act as a source of peritoneal infection.

# GYNECOLOGICAL AND OBSTETRICAL TUBERCULOSIS

CHARLES C. NORRIS, M.D.

## APPENDIX

### TUBERCULOSIS OF THE KIDNEY

Tuberculosis of the kidney occurs in two distinct forms: (*a*) as a part of the general miliary tuberculosis and (*b*) the so-called primary renal tuberculosis. The renal involvement is generally of comparatively minor importance in the first variety. This type is not included in the following study.

Renal tuberculosis is practically always secondary. The primary lesion may be small, quiescent, and difficult or impossible to recognize clinically. The fact that the condition is secondary and a part only of a general infection, has an important bearing upon the prognosis and treatment.

Much advance has been made in recent years in methods of diagnosis and treatment, and the knowledge that chronic renal tuberculosis is always a surgical disease is now recognized. Medical treatment alone is rarely, if ever, successful, but combined with proper surgical procedure, is of the utmost importance.

Renal tuberculosis still presents many unsolved problems. The pathologic changes incident to early renal tuberculosis have been studied experimentally but are still somewhat in doubt. The fact that early renal tuberculosis gives rise to no symptoms or only vague clinical manifestations is regrettable, and it is to be hoped that in the future a method may be developed which will enable recognition during the incipiency of the disease.

As has been intimated, the term primary renal tuberculosis is generally employed in a clinical rather than etiological sense. Morgagni and other writers described renal tuberculosis but the mode of infection was misunderstood. Prior to the surgical era the disease was generally described by the pathologists who saw advanced bilateral lesions with extensive vesical involvement and often invasion of other organs. The condition was thought incurable. Probably owing to the prominence of the vesical symptom it was believed that the infection was an ascending one. In 1871 Simon, by the performance of nephrectomy, did much to stimulate the successful treatment of renal tuberculosis. The period between 1878 and 1893 saw great improvement in the methods of diagnosis and during the last decade of the twentieth century the operation of nephrectomy was perfected and became widely employed.

**Etiology.**—Renal tuberculosis is usually caused by the human variety of the tubercle bacillus. The bovine tubercle bacillus is of less frequent occurrence. In the early stages of the disease the condition is generally due to the tubercle bacillus alone, but in the later stages mixed infection, particularly with the colon bacillus and the ordinary pyogenic organisms, is of frequent occurrence.

Various conditions have been thought to be predisposing factors to renal tuberculosis; among the most commonly assigned being ptosis, hydronephrosis, renal calculus, pregnancy, heredity, acute nephritis, chronic nephritis, gonorrhea, trauma, congenital malformations, chronic pyelitis, cystitis, urethritis, hypernephroma and any condition that produces urinary stasis, such as hypertrophy of prostate, stricture, and allied conditions.

PTOSIS.—It has been suggested that kinking of the ureter, increase in intrarenal pressure and interference with the circulation of the kidney, may be predisposing factors. However, clinical studies do not bear out this assertion. Renal ptosis is much more common in the female than in the male, but whereas statistical studies do show a greater frequency of renal tuberculosis in the female, the proportion is not marked.

HYDRONEPHROSIS.—It is doubtful what part hydronephrosis plays as a predisposing factor to infection by tuberculosis. Stasis and intrarenal changes in pressure are, theoretically at least, causative factors. From a practical standpoint it is often difficult to determine whether or not the hydronephrosis actually preceded the tuberculosis or was the result of it.

PREGNANCY.—Renal tuberculosis in association with pregnancy is not infrequent. It is recognized that pregnancy often produces an exacerbation of previously quiescent tuberculous lesions, especially those in the lungs, and that a bacillemia not infrequently results. It also frequently produces a stasis and renal congestion. All these are factors which would appear to favor a renal involvement.

HEREDITY.—Renal tuberculosis is most common in middle life. Undoubtedly there is a predisposition to tuberculosis in general, but the part played by it in the production of renal tuberculosis is probably slight.

ACUTE AND CHRONIC NEPHRITIS.—That acute and chronic nephritis are predisposing factors to renal tuberculosis rests only upon theoretic grounds.

GONORRHEA.—Gonorrheal pyelitis is such a rare condition as to be almost negligible as far as being an important predisposing factor in renal tuberculosis. Preëxisting gonorrheal infection is probably a definite predisposing factor to tuberculous salpingitis and it is probably a predisposing factor in the kidney.

TRAUMA.—In some instances trauma has apparently played a predisposing part in the development of renal tuberculosis. Owing to its protected location the kidney is rarely exposed to this insult. Experimental research apparently indicates that trauma acts as a predisposing cause.

CONGENITAL MALFORMATION.—A study of a large series of cases seems to show that tuberculosis is more frequently in kidneys the seat of a congenital malformation, especially of the lobulated variety. This is in accord with the findings regarding tuberculosis elsewhere in the body.

It is generally stated that tuberculosis of the kidney may be primary or secondary and may result from an ascending or descending infection, or in rare instances from direct extension from adjacent foci. A few cases of apparently true primary renal tuberculosis are on record. Opinions differ regarding the existence of even these and many close observers believe that this is never the case.

Certainly true primary lesions are extremely rare and are of interest from a theoretic rather than a practical standpoint. All cases should be treated as if secondary. The infection is usually hematogenous and descending in type. Occasionally infection may occur via the lymphatics. The infection may be an ascending one by way of the urogenital system and may occur by continuity from adjacent foci such as tuberculosis of the adrenals, spine, pleura, intestines, peritoneum, etc. It is at least theoretically possible that the old theory of ascension from the bladder via the ureter or peri-ureteral lymphatics may occasionally occur. Brown (Brown, T. R. Osler's *Modern Medicine.* 1919, Vol. VI. 274) points out that many cases have been regarded as ascending infection because of the advanced development of the lesions in the papillæ, the pelvis, or the ureter, but this argument is fallacious because the changes in the medulla are often secondary to some primary focus in the cortex, although the medullary lesion may develop more rapidly, affect the renal pelvis and ureter, and produce the appearance of greater age. It is also quite possible for a hematogenous infection to be primary in the pyramids or pelvis.

Primary vesical tuberculosis is extremely rare. Young (Young, H. *Phila. Urol. Soc.* Jan. 26, 1925) states that he has never seen a case. The true primary focus of renal tuberculosis is most commonly pulmonary or intestinal and less frequently from the lymphatic glands, fallopian tube, or osseous system.

The passage of tubercle bacilli through the kidney without causing a lesion is important. It is well known that the mere demonstration of tubercle bacilli in the urine is insufficient evidence upon which to base the diagnosis of genito-urinary tuberculosis. Cunningham, Brown,

Crabtree, and others have reported such occurrences. It has been found that tubercle bacilli are sometimes secreted in the urine in cases of pulmonary tuberculosis in which there is no demonstrable renal lesion. Whereas the presence of tubercle bacilli in the urine is strong presumptive evidence of urogenital tuberculosis, unless pus and other evidence is also present, it is not conclusive. The presence of predisposing factors, the number and virulence of the tubercle bacilli reaching the kidney, the local and general resistance of the individual, are probably the determining points as to whether or not a renal infection develops in these cases.

**Pathology.**—The methods by which the tubercle bacillus may reach the kidney have been enumerated. There is nothing in the macroscopic or histologic study of renal tuberculosis which will with certainty determine the mode of infection nor can the initial renal lesion be positively differentiated. Experimental evidence which is confirmed by histologic and clinical study, however, shows that generally the tubercle-bearing emboli find lodgment between the cortex and medulla near the base of a pyramid. Crabtree (Crabtree, E. G. Cabot's *Modern Urology*. 1924, Vol. II. 530) states that most of the tubercle bacilli which reach the kidney through the renal artery, are arrested in glomeruli. Some few escape from the capillaries of the glomeruli by the efferent blood stream and may be enmeshed in the complex venous channels which surround the tubules or descend with them toward the pelvis. They may also lodge in the area supplied by the arterioles originating directly from the renal artery.

Many classifications of renal tuberculosis have been made. Israel divides the lesions into three groups: (*a*) phthisis caseosa, often associated with peri- and paranephritis and frequently developing into pyonephrosis; (*b*) ulcerations of the tips of the papillæ, less frequent but often productive of hematuria; and (*c*) a chronic disseminated variety somewhat resembling the acute miliary type except that the disease is unilateral and the tubercles larger and necrosis and caseation more definite. Proliferation of the epithelium and endothelial cells are characteristic and early changes. The degree of small round cell infiltration is variable. In the center of the tubercles fat formation occurs, followed by breaking down of the cells. Tubercle bacilli can be demonstrated in the tubercules and are most common near the periphery. The pathologic picture varies with the duration of the disease. Specimens may be observed in which the lesion is limited to a few small tubercles and vary from this to destruction of the entire kidney and involvement of adjacent structures.

The disease is a progressive one. The most commonly observed macroscopic picture in specimens removed by operation is one or more small caseous areas, a centimeter or more in diameter. This is most often in a pyramid. The caseous area contains flaky, greenish or yellowish pus and the wall is shaggy. Often one lesion is considerably larger than another. These lesions are generally buried in the substance of the kidney but may project under the capsule. The ureter is usually thickened and as the disease advances, the caseous areas increase in size and one or more may coalesce so that it is not uncommon to find one pole of the kidney entirely occupied by such a lesion. In advanced cases the entire renal tissue may be destroyed and the kidney converted into an abscess sac surrounded by the capsule, which, even in advanced cases, tends to retain its integrity.

Tuffier has described a form of massive degeneration combined with occlusion of the ureter in which the entire kidney is destroyed and but little enlarged. As a general rule considerable enlargement is present in the advanced stages. When the renal pelvis is involved the mucosa is reddened, thickened, roughened, has lost its sheen and may show more or less definite ulceration in varying degrees, which is likely to be on the lateral aspects of the papillæ. Tubercles may be demonstrable macroscopically.

In the early cases the cortex appears normal but may contain macroscopic tubercles. In the later stages, the so-called ulcerocavernous type, the kidney is generally enlarged, congested, and a collection of tubercles is often visible beneath the capsule. More or less extensive ulceration is present, especially of the papillæ; adhesions to the capsule and about the pelvis are common. When the cortex is involved, adhesions to the fatty capsule may be extensive.

If obstruction of the ureter occurs a pyonephrosis follows. The organ is generally enlarged and lobulated; the kidney tissue is thinned. Not infrequently pyonephrosis develops, even when no obstruction can be demonstrated, and has been accounted for by disease of the walls of the pelvis and ureter, which become lax and dilate easily. Loss of tone appears to be the cause in some of these cases; occasionally, in extremely advanced cases, the entire kidney is destroyed, the ureter completely blocked, the blood supply shut off, and the contents of the capsule becomes thickened and inspissated with calcium salts producing a light-grayish putty-like material.

This condition has been termed autonephrectomy. Even such "dead" kidneys have been found to contain virulent tubercle bacilli. Occasionally specimens are encountered which contain more or less cicatricial tissues, apparently the result of an attempt by nature to cure the condition. Active lesions are always present in these kidneys, which are often small and adherent. Crabtree terms them sclerous tuberculosis.

Much has been written, especially by the earlier writers, concerning spontaneous healing of renal tuberculosis. The writer has never seen such a specimen, and a moderately extensive search through the literature has failed to reveal an authentic case. This is of importance in regard to the treatment. The fact that active, although often microscopic tubercles are present, even in kidneys in which attempts at healing are evident, is the strongest argument against nephrotomy or resection of a part of the kidney.

When tuberculosis develops in a malformed kidney of the double type, one pelvis is generally macroscopically invaded, and the cortical portion of the other organ often contains microscopic evidence of infection.

The histologic picture produced in tuberculosis of the kidney is in general similar to that resulting from a like infection elsewhere. The tubercle bacillus is generally arrested in the glomerula near the medulla and tubercles develop at this point. The amount of chronic inflammation is variable and often not marked even in advanced cases. The tubercles develop, coalesce, and form nodules which undergo caseation, which in turn is probably due to the toxins produced by the tubercle bacillus.

The toxins injure the cells in which fatty changes occur. This is followed by death and disintegration of these structures. Calcium from the blood stream is deposited, and leads to chemical changes which are said to result in the formation of calcium soap from the combination of fatty acids.

The larger tubercles may be distinguished macroscopically as grayish, whitish, or yellowish areas with softened centers. These may be discrete and scattered through the medulla or cortex, but more frequently coalesce forming cavities of varying size. When the pelvis of the kidney is invaded and there is free drainage, there is generally less enlargement of the kidney than when obstruction occurs.

Obstruction usually occurs sooner or later and in most instances of moderate advancement more or less enlargement of the kidney is present.

When involvement of the pelvis has occurred, the ureter becomes infected, tubercles form, followed by caseation and ulceration; the ureter becomes thickened and infiltrated, and in a short time bladder involvement develops by direct extension from the ureter. Stricture of the ureter or entire occlusion of the ureteral lumen may occur, or the lumen become temporarily blocked by detritus. Dilatation and stricture is common in advanced cases. In specimens of renal tuberculosis removed by nephrectomy the ureter is nearly always involved and in postmortem specimens, almost routinely.

When secondary infection by pyogenic organism takes place, the symptoms are intensified; active, inflammatory reactions occur, and the kidney may be converted into a huge abscess sac with little or no renal tissue remaining. With the addition of pyogenic organism the integrity of the capsule is prone to be destroyed, and perinephritic abscesses result. Perinephritic abscesses are much more likely to develop when mixed infection occurs than when the tubercle bacillus is the only organism present. In some specimens there is a predominance of scar tissue in the fibrous capsule and the surrounding fat or typical tuberculous lesion may be observed.

Tuberculosis of the ureter and bladder is nearly always secondary to renal tuberculosis. When the renal pelvis becomes involved, a descending infection follows, and the symptoms resulting from this are generally more marked than those produced by the kidney lesion. Fortunately, the ureteral and vesical lesions tend to heal after nephrectomy. The infection is by contiguity and extends along the submucosa; from here extending to the muscularis and peri-ureteral tissue and to the mucosa.

In advanced cases the fat surrounding the pelvis contains tubercles. As might be expected from a descending infection, vesical tuberculosis develops primarily about the ureteral opening, which is reddened and swollen and may show macroscopic ulcers or macroscopic tubercles.

The chief vesical lesion is about the ureteral opening, but from here the disease may spread and in advanced cases invade the entire bladder. The apparent immunity of the bladder to the action of the tubercle bacillus is remarkable, and even in advanced cases observed at necropsy, the ureteral orifices and adjacent bladder walls are often the only areas affected. This is in accord with the rarity of so-called primary vesical tuberculosis. The characteristic appearance of vesical tuberculosis is of the utmost value in the cystoscopic examination.

Except in the miliary variety, renal tuberculosis is nearly always unilateral in its incipiency, and generally it is only in the late stages that the opposite kidney is involved. The route by which the second kidney becomes infected is somewhat in doubt. Metastasis from the primary affected kidney, ureter or bladder, or from the true primary focus has been suggested. Naturally, statistics vary widely regarding the frequency with which the second kidney is involved and depend largely upon the type of material utilized. Postmortem records show a high proportion of bilateral renal tuberculosis whereas those formulated from operative material present the reverse aspect. Halle and Morz (*Ann. d. mal. d. org. genito-urin.*, Par. 1906. 24:241) in necropsy material found 42 of 131 cases of renal tuberculosis to be bilateral.

Brown (Brown, T. E. *loc. cit.*) quotes from Douglas, Bevan, Albarran, Morabeau, Krönlein, Israel, Krummel, Flackman, and Kuster, whose combined statistics show unilateral lesions in 83.66 per cent. Other authorities present even more favorable figures. The experience of the writer is that at least 90 per cent of cases are unilateral that come for operation provided that ordinary diagnostic skill has been exercised in the recognition of the condition.

When bilateral, renal tuberculosis is present similar types of lesions are usually observed. However, one kidney nearly always shows greater advancement of the disease. Numerous cases of renal tuberculosis occurring in conjunction with calculi have been analyzed but it is questionable if the percentage of such cases is greater than could be accounted for by the disease incident of the condition. Generally the stone precedes the tuberculosis and upon theoretic grounds at least may be supposed to be a predisposing factor to the latter.

Walker (*Ann. Surg.* 1907. 14: 249, 388, 597) in a series of 218 cases found the right kidney diseased in 111, and the left in 98; in nine the affected side was not stated. These figures closely approximate those given by most observers.

Chronic renal tuberculosis may lead to a toxic nephritis of the opposite kidney which generally clears up promptly after nephrectomy. In some cases this is entirely a functional condition; in others, particularly those of long standing, a chronic parenchymatous nephritis develops with its usual symptoms of urinary findings. A comparative degree of compensatory hypertrophy in the normal kidney is prone to occur.

**Symptoms.**—Statistics are quite variable in regard to the bearing which sex plays in the development of renal tuberculosis. G. Walker's series (*loc. cit.*), in 386 patients, 204 were females. In the same series the average age was 27.66 years. In our much smaller series the average age was 35 years. The disease is therefore most frequent in adult life.

Although pregnancy frequently exerts an unfavorable influence on pulmonary tuberculosis and results in an exacerbation and tuberculous bacteriemia, child bearing apparently plays no appreciable part in the development of renal lesions and the disease is relatively as frequent at least in small series, in the nulliparous as in the multiparous. A family history of tuberculosis or of exposure to the infection is frequent but may be absent. Careful questioning will often elicit a history suggestive of tuberculosis elsewhere in the body; a history of susceptibility to "colds," pleurisy, chronic lung lesions, chronic abscesses, persistent sinuses, adenitis or even of chronic peritonitis is not infrequent. A thorough examination of the lungs should be made by an experienced internist in every case.

The clinical evidence of a true active primary lesion is often lacking at the time of the development of the renal symptoms. Indeed it is not uncommon in cases of renal tuberculosis to be unable to determine the true primary focus. Renal tuberculosis in its early stages produces few and mild symptoms, and this is unfortunate, as the earlier the diagnosis can be established and nephrectomy performed, the better is the prognosis. A thorough investigation will often show that for some time the patient has been below par, that there has been malaise, poor appetite, a feeling of warmth or feverishness, especially in the late afternoons or evenings, and poor sleep.

In the early stages of the disease, constitutional symptoms vary markedly in different cases but are generally absent or so insignificant as to escape notice. Fever was present in but 22 per cent of Israel's cases of uncomplicated renal tuberculosis and in 80 per cent of those in which the bladder was involved. After extensive caseous areas have developed or in the presence of a mixed infection, hyperexia is generally the rule. A slight evening rise of temperature is always significant; loss of weight, anemia, hyperexia, exhausting sweats, and other evidence of toxemias are late symptoms. Digestive disturbance, nausea, vomiting, diarrhea, constipation, anorexia, rapidity of the pulse, anemia, may occur early but are generally of late occurrence. Pain depends upon the stage and type of lesion present. In the early stages it is almost a negligible symptom. Hypotension has been observed and thought to be of value as a diagnostic sign.

Tenderness over the region of the kidney is of frequent occurrence and may develop moderately early. Later when the ureter is affected tenderness in that structure is generally present. Palpation of the ureter in its lower portion and especially as it crosses the pelvic brim and as it passes through the paramentrium to enter the bladder, as elicited by a vaginal examination, is a valuable diagnostic symptom. The thickened and cordlike ureter may often be palpated by this method. Such ureters are sometimes referred to as pipestem or rosary-like, according to whether the thickening is uniform or nodular.

Crossed or referred pain may develop. This is a pain which occurs in the uninfected kidney; it is the result of swelling or compensatory hypertrophy of the kidney and consequent stretching of its capsule. It is prone to occur in rapidly advancing cases, and in those in which there is obstruction to the outflow on the affected side. It is of importance in that pain in the supposedly normal kidney does not necessarily infer a bilateral infection. The pain in the affected kidney is generally of a dull aching character or may be only a feeling of pressure. As obstruction begins colicky attacks develop, generally in the affected area but sometimes referred along the course of the ureter. When vesical involvement is marked the thickened bladder can be easily felt upon bimanual examination. When the bladder becomes affected dysuria and frequency become prominent symptoms and are usually at first most marked at night. Vesical irritation is often the first symptom which induces the patient to seek medical aid. Such symptoms should never be overlooked or treated empirically until a thorough investigation of the case has been made. It cannot be too strongly emphasized that not infrequently these are the first severe symptoms from which the patient complains and the possibility of a tuberculous nephritis being present should always be borne in mind by the attending physician.

In not a few cases the diagnosis of uncomplicated cystitis is made and the true nature of the condition not recognized until the disease is hopelessly advanced. Some writers, recognizing the mildness of the early symptoms resulting from renal tuberculosis, divide the disease into four stages: (1) early, when symptoms are absent or almost silent, (2) involvement of the pyramids and ureter, (3) the vesical stage, and (4) when bilateral infection has occurred. As has been intimated, the symptoms vary widely with the individual case and with the stage of the disease. As a rule the diagnosis is not easy or may be impossible in the early stage and is generally quite apparent during the later development of the condition. Palpation will generally show some tenderness even in the early stage of the disease; later the kidney may be enlarged, especially if obstruction has occurred. Enlargement of the kidney is more easily recognized upon the right than on the left side. In about one half the cases coming to operation the enlargement of the kidney can be recognized by palpation. Definite local swelling is generally indicative of hydronephrosis, pyonephrosis or paranephritic abscess.

Leukocytosis is generally absent unless a mixed infection is present. Renal tuberculosis usually runs a chronic but progressively unfavorable course. Remission of symptoms may occur for varying periods, especially in the early stages of the disease and sometimes leads to the fallacious hope that the condition has been caused by medical treatment, or in the unrecognized cases, that local applications to a supposed cystitis have proved effectual. These remissions are caused by the free drainage of a hitherto troublesome caseous area and comparative freedom from symptoms continue until new lesions develop or a light-up of the earlier area occurs. The remission of symptoms both local and general are characteristic of renal tuberculosis; intervals of entire absence of pain, gain in weight and absence of renal symptoms are of frequent occurrence.

Tuberculosis of the kidney may develop during the course of pregnancy, or pregnancy may occur during the course of a renal tuberculosis. There is little doubt that pregnancy exerts an unfavorable influence on the course of the disease. Not only is this true of tuberculosis in general, but in these cases the congestion produced by the pregnancy and the added strain which is thrown on the kidneys incident to gestation, act deleteriously.

It is unwise to attempt anything but generalities regarding the treatment of the pregnant tuberculous woman. In the early stages of pregnancy complicated by renal tuberculosis, therapeutic abortion is often indicated. Whether or not this should be done should depend upon the condition of the patient and the advancement of the renal lesion. At all events the nephrectomy should not be delayed on account of the pregnancy and the emptying of the uterus is generally advisable.

If it is decided to terminate the pregnancy, the same methods advised in the chapter on Pulmonary Tuberculosis and Pregnancy are advisable. Very early pregnancy may be successfully interrupted by dilatation and the use of placental forceps. From the sixth week on, however, vaginal hysterectomy, especially in the multipara, and when the cervix can be brought well down, is the method of choice.

This operation may be quickly performed. There is little loss of blood and convalescence is generally extremely rapid and smooth, and is uncomplicated by bleeding and the necessity for repeated uterine packing. It can be performed at the same time as the nephrectomy, if the condition of the patient warrants the slight prolongation of anesthesia incident to the procedure.

More or less the same advice holds true from the fourth to the sixth or seventh month; as the nephrectomy itself may produce abortion or premature labor, this consideration should be borne in mind. Towards the end of pregnancy it may be advisable to delay the nephrectomy a few weeks in the interest of the child, but as a general rule the pregnancy should be disregarded and the renal tuberculosis treated as if pregnancy did not exist. If there is hope of saving the chiid gradual dilatation of the cervix may be resorted to and the nephrectomy and delivery by forceps or version performed jointly.

Subsequent to nephrectomy for tuberculosis, it is generally inadvisable for patients to become pregnant. No hard and fast rules should, however, be formulated. It should be remembered that, entirely apart from the added burden on the remaining kidney incident to pregnancy, these patients are tuberculous, and even though the focus is quiescent, the physiologic changes incident to pregnancy may be sufficient to produce an exacerbation.

Borelius (Borelius, R. *Monatschr. f. Geburtsh. u. Gynaek.* 1924. 67: 327-393) reports the results in cases of pregnancy after nephrectomy. He believes there is no evidence of increased frequency of abortions after nephrectomy and that an existing pregnancy does not contraindicate nephrectomy.

Urinary Symptoms.—As already stated, not infrequently the first indication of the presence of renal tuberculosis is frequency, urgency, dysuria, polyuria, pyuria, hematuria, and symptoms suggestive of vesical irritability. Frequency is the most commonly observed symptom. Especially in advanced cases, vesical irritability is marked, and tortures the patient day and night, making life almost unendurable. Roberts has recorded the history of a patient who voided 180 times daily and in whom the bladder was only slightly involved.

Pyuria, sometimes intermittent, due to blockage, is a symptom of the utmost importance. Frequency and pyuria, especially in conjunction with a comparatively normal bladder, is especially significant. Patients often notice the cloudy appearance of the urine and remark upon its changes from day to day. The pus from a tuberculous kidney is grayish and granular and gives the urine a ground-glass appearance in contrast to the soft yellowish pus produced by most other conditions. As caseation advances in the open lesion, pyuria becomes marked and as fragments of the detritus produce blockage, colic develops, sometimes not unlike that caused by a calculus. If the blockage is complete or other occlusions of the ureter develop, there will be a temporary cessation of the pyuria or a marked lessening of the amount of pus. A small amount of pus may be present in the urine, due to lesions below the point of blockage. Naturally, much depends upon the stage of the disease and the character of the renal lesion as well as upon the condition of the ureter and bladder. The presence of pyuria, at least in the early stage, depends upon whether the lesion involves the pelvis or calices. Large quantities of purulent material in the urine generally indicate that a mixed infection is present.

Hematuria or a few red blood corpuscles in combination with pyuria is of frequent occurrence and is an important symptom. Macroscopic hematuria may be present especially if the apices of the papillæ are involved. Macroscopic and even microscopic hematuria tends to be intermittent. Sometimes clots produce blockage and colic and complete casts of the ureter have been observed. Occasionally macroscopic hematuria is the first symptom. Cases have been recorded in which no blood has been demonstrable in the urine. Polyuria is present in many cases and may be intermittent in type. The urine is of a low specific gravity. Albuminuria in correspondence with the amount of pus or blood or due to an associated nephritis is present. Casts are often lacking. They were observed in 10 per cent of Hunner's cases. Hyaline and granular casts are the most frequent.

Casts are indicative of a nephritis; they may have their origin in the non-tuberculous kidney. The urine is acid in all stages of renal tuberculosis, unless vesical involvement is present, or a mixed infection has occurred. Hence in the early stages it is nearly always acid. Particles of cheesy material, friable detritus, elastic fibers, are of frequent occurrence in the urine. Incomplete retention and spasmodic incontinence may occur. In tuberculosis of the kidney the bladder urine may be sterile in ordinary culture media, even though considerable pus is present. This is itself is a suggestive sign of tuberculous nephritis. A mixed infection may be misleading and tend to obscure the correct diagnosis.

The demonstration of tubercle bacillus in the urine is the most important single symptom in the diagnosis of renal tuberculosis. That it is not absolutely diagnostic, however, has already been stated, as in certain conditions tubercle bacillus may be passed through the normal kidney. The presence of tubercle bacilli and pus in specimens secured by ureteral catheterization is however conclusive. The importance of the test for these organisms is therefore apparent. The tubercle bacillus must be differentiated from the smegma bacillus which is morphologically and tinctorially nearly similar.

The most certain method of demonstrating the tubercle bacillus is by guinea-pig inoculation but this has the disadvantage of being time-consuming, and although the Block method considerably shortens this period, the necessary wait incident to even this procedure may be inadvisable. Whatever method of diagnosis is employed, animal inoculation should always be performed and a number of animals should be utilized. It is unsafe to rely upon a single or even two animals. An accidental infection may occur or a single pig may die shortly after inoculation.

Loewenstein in 1913 and later Hyntschak (Hyntschak, I. *Wien. klin. Wchnschr.* 1924. 37:336) have pointed out that renal tuberculosis may result from the tubercle bacillus of fowls and that this organism is not pathogenic to guinea pigs. These authors emphasize the importance of cultures by the Loewenstein method. Various cultural methods have been suggested for the demonstration of the tubercle bacillus, chief among them is that of Brown and Petroeff mentioned in a preceding chapter. A reliable cultural method would be of great value.

Barney, quoted by Cabot, states (*Modern Urology.* 1914. Vol. II, 552) the value of the animal test cannot be doubted and is well shown by a series of 252 consecutive pig inoculations done at the Massachusetts General Hospital; of these 197 were definitely proved either positive or negative by operation, pathologic report, and autopsy or clinical course. Among these were two cases in which the pathologic report showed tuberculosis of the kidney and the pig test was negative. In one of these there was complete obliteration of the ureter. In the other there was a tuberculous nephritic abscess but the pig test was negative. Leaving out the first of these cases the pig test was accurate in 99.5 per cent of the 197 cases.

It is a good practice to look for tubercle bacillus in every acid, apparently sterile, purulent urine as well as in all cases which present other suggestive symptoms. Bladder urine may be employed for animal inoculation. Tubercle bacillus may be demonstrated by staining methods from the bladder urine but the dangers of contamination, especially by the smegma bacillus, must be considered. In specimens secured by aseptically performed vesical catheterization the danger of contamination by the smegma bacillus is considerably lessened. The dangers of contamination by the smegma bacillus are somewhat greater in the female than in the male. The 24-hour specimens are, however, more difficult to secure by this method. Urine secured by properly performed ureteral catheterization is almost sure to be uncontaminated, but the small amount obtainable is sometimes a detrimental factor. If tubercle bacillus and pus can be demonstrated in such urine by staining methods it is practically convincing proof of the existence of renal tuberculosis.

Ureteral catheterization should be employed in every suspicious case as well as the examination of the 24-hour specimen. Properly performed ureteral catheterization is practically devoid of danger and certainly is productive of less risk than that incurred by failure to perform the operation and subsequent delay and doubtful results by other methods. It must be remembered that at times tubercle bacillus may be absent from the urine or present only in extremely small numbers, especially in the early stages of the disease, and that the failure to demonstrate the organisms by a single examination does not exclude the possibility of tuberculosis being present. Repeated tests should be made in suspicious cases. However, a competent bacteriologist will rarely fail to detect the tubercle bacillus if present. Cabot (*Modern Urology*. 1924, Vol. II, 552) states that at the Massachusetts General Hospital they have been strong believers in the accuracy of the guinea-pig test and until recently have relied upon it entirely.

Autonephrectomy, obliteration, and blockage of the ureter may at times produce periods when the tubercle bacillus may be temporarily or permanently absent from the urine.

**Cystoscopic Examination and Ureteral Catheterization.**—Modern cystoscopy is one of the most valuable methods in the diagnosis of renal tuberculosis and has revolutionized the methods of diagnosis. Not only is it an aid to diagnosis but the procedure offers a method by which the extent of the disease may be determined in the majority of cases. The various separators or segregators are unreliable.

Even in the hands of the experienced cystoscopist the cystoscopic examination and ureteral catheterization is not entirely without risk but this risk is extremely small. The perforation of a tuberculous bladder or ureter has been recorded. A suspected case, however, runs a far greater risk from delay than from the prompt employment of this method.

If marked vesical irritability is present the exhibition of sandalwood 0.9 c.c. for a few days prior to the cystoscopic examination may be beneficial together with the ingestion of a considerable extra quantity of water. In this connection it should be remembered that hexamethylenetetramin and its derivatives are often irritating in renal tuberculosis.

It is of great advantage to complete the cystoscopic examination at one sitting. Anesthesia is not generally necessary. A weak novocaine may be employed if necessary. In nervous women morphine sulphate (grn. ¼) may be given hypodermically half an hour before the examination. A general anesthetic is neither required nor advisable and hinders the examination in many respects. Cabot (*loc. cit.*) has occasionally employed spinal anesthesia.

The bladder should be thoroughly washed out as a preliminary step. The appearance of the bladder is often characteristic. In early cases it may appear normal. The ureteral orifice of the affected side generally appears reddened and swollen and tubercles may be seen as small grayish elevations surrounded by a reddened base. The tubercles exhibit a tendency to break down, resulting in irregular shallow ulcers, to which may be attached cheesy-like material. The trigone is often edematous or may be definitely involved in the tuberculous process. Extensive tuberculous trigonitis is, however, unusual and rarely observed except in advanced cases. Due to infiltration, the action of the ureteral sphincter is sluggish. When the ureter is extensively involved its orifice tends to retract, due to thickening and edema. There may or may not be an associated ulcer. Sometimes this retraction is so marked that the affected ureteral orifice appears in the midline.

From inspection the experienced cystoscopist is often able to arrive at the diagnosis. It is needless to add this diagnosis should be verified by other means. Ureteral catheterization should be performed not only to determine the condition of both kidneys but to ascertain the condition of the ureters. The separate urines should be subjected to a rigid study.

It is essential to determine the condition of both kidneys. If one ureteral orifice is obviously diseased and the other appears normal it is generally better to catheterize only the apparently normal side. In advanced cases of tuberculous ureteritis, strictures, distortions or other abnormalities are prone to be present which may prevent the passage of a catheter, or the ureter may be so dilated that the urine escapes around the instrument. If the bladder and ureteral orifices are normal, or any doubt exists as to which is the affected side, both ureters must be catheterized. The same is true if both appear involved.

Ureteral catheterization, while most valuable, is not without its hazards. The risk of carrying infected material from the bladder into a normal ureter, or even to the kidney, must be considered. This danger may be almost entirely eliminated by proper technic. To obtain renal urine it is not necessary to pass the catheter all the way to the kidney; a few centimeters are sufficient. Constitutional and local symptoms may follow even properly performed ureteral catheterization and a certain amount of malaise and discomfort is of frequent occurrence. The risk when proper technic is employed is at the minimum. The benefits to be derived from the method far outweigh its risks. Only by ureteral catheterization is it possible to determine with certainty the condition of the supposedly normal kidney and in other cases ascertain which side is affected.

As a general rule ureteral catheterization presents no particular difficulties, when the bladder is extensively involved, markedly edematous or ulcerated or when much cicatricial tissue is present even the experienced cystoscopist may have difficulty in locating the ureteral openings. Chromatocystoscopy may be resorted to. It takes 10 to 15 minutes for the coloring matter to appear, and this is a distinct disadvantage if the bladder is irritable, as it is likely to be in the type of case in which chromatocystoscopy is required. However this disadvantage may be largely overcome by careful timing. The chromatocystoscopic part of the examination should be performed prior to the insertion of the ureteral catheterization, as the latter procedure may produce a ureteral spasm which is detrimental to the accuracy of the test. At the risk of repetition we would emphasize the importance of concluding all the cystoscopic work at one sitting. Tuberculous bladders are generally irritable and for this reason it is important to work as rapidly as compatible with thoroughness and to have no delays between the various steps in the examination. With this in view, the examination should be performed in a well-equipped cystoscopic room, aided by an assistant and a well-trained nurse. In cases of doubtful diagnosis Buerger has performed biopsy through the cystoscope and in this way has been able to establish a diagnosis.

The functional tests are of value in determining the condition of the supposedly normal kidney as well as the diseased one. Double ureters and other anomalies must be looked for. One remarkable specimen of this condition occurred upon the gynecological service at the University Hospital, in which the urine from one ureter was normal and from the other showed the usual evidence of tuberculosis.

**Diagnosis.**—In the early stage the diagnosis is often difficult and the lesion nearly silent. A careful review of most cases will, however, often show that some suggestive symptom has been present, even in the early stage, and in the preceding pages an endeavor has been made to emphasize the importance of these symptoms. All cases presenting suggestive symptoms should be subject to a thorough and, if necessary, repeated examination. Negative urine findings are not uncommon in the incipiency of the disease and this is the type of cases in which a second or even a third cystoscopic examination is required. As the bladders in this stage are not likely to be irritable there is less objection to a second cystoscopic examination in this class of patient than in those with more pronounced lesions. During the later stages of the disease its recognition is generally easy.

X-ray examinations are of great value in arriving at a diagnosis and in excluding renal calculus. Calcified areas may simulate calculi. Tuberculous lesions appear denser than normal renal tissue. The amount of involvement is often determinable, to an extent at least, by the x-ray. The tuberculin test is employed by some urologists. The general reaction is of little value in the adult but the local reaction of pain in the renal area is suggestive. Renal functional tests are of much importance and one of these should be employed in every case. The phenolsulphonephthalein test is one of the best; the divided as well as the total function may be estimated. Probably the best plan is to employ both the phenolsulphonephthalein and indigo-carmine tests. Both can be utilized at one sitting. This combination gives a most accurate estimate. The conditions for which renal tuberculosis is likely to be mistaken are pyelitis, cystic kidney, calculus, hypernephroma and other malignant neoplasms, and essential hematuria. Calculi and neoplasms are most likely to cause confusion, but can be readily differentiated if proper means or employed. Having established the diagnosis no time should be lost in instituting treatment.

In rare instances when some insurmountable obstacle exists, such as ankylosis of the hip joints, stricture, etc., it may be advisable to make a vesicovaginal fistula and catheterize the ureters through the opening, or even to perform an extraperitoneal exploration of the kidney.

**Treatment.**—The only satisfactory treatment for renal tuberculosis is nephrectomy. This operation is indicated in all cases as soon as the diagnosis is established provided the disease is unilateral, that the functional tests shows the opposite kidney in good condition and supposing no other contraindications such as an advanced pulmonary tuberculosis are present. Watson and Cunningham (*Genito-Urinary Diseases.* Phila. & N. Y., 1908. Vol. II. 400) emphasize the importance of establishing the functional capability of the kidney which is to remain after the removal of its fellow by their collected statistics. In the first series which numbers 362, the tests of the functional capability of the other kidney were not made; the operative mortality was 35 per cent. In the second series the tests were employed and the operative mortality was 7.8 per cent.

The presence of active tuberculous lesions elsewhere in the body is not an absolute contra-indication to operation. It must be remembered that if the kidney is not removed the patient will die, and considerable risks are therefore justifiable. Cases must be judged individually. Active lesions often improve after operation. Sometimes a short course of carefully instituted treatment will convert an active lesion into one safely permitting operation. Every case is surgical unless surgery is contraindicated. In the vast literature which has accumulated regarding the treatment of renal tuberculosis, there are but a few cases in which it is claimed medical treatment alone has effected a cure. Even these are open to doubt. In years past even the most ardent advocate of the nonsurgical treatment claimed results in only the early cases and were there no difficulty in definitely discriminating between the very early cases and the moderately advanced, the fact that nephrectomy is associated with such a small mortality and gives such excellent results in these early cases, is a sufficient reason for urging operation in every case.

The essentials for a satisfactory operation are a long incision, which facilitates the procedure and permits the removal of the kidney without rupture, and the excision of as much of the upper portion of the ureter as can be removed without unduly complicating the operation. It has been found that a tuberculous ureter and bladder will undergo complete resuscitation in nearly all cases after nephrectomy. Some surgeons have recommended complete ureterectomy in conjunction with nephrectomy. The removal of the entire ureter necessitates greatly prolonging the operation, and is inadvisable largely because of the operative difficulties, combined with the fact that practice has amply demonstrated these lesions undergo resolution. It is therefore useless and not worth the additional risk incurred by its performance. The only cases which may require complete ureterectomy are those in which a stricture exists in the lower portion of the ureter, which prevents subsequent drainage. Even this may generally be overcome by dilatation.

Care in not contaminating the wound and absolute hemostasis are essential. An extraperitoneal operation should be performed. Under such circumstances, closure without drainage is the most satisfactory procedure. If doubt exists as to this point, or if the patient is fat, a small wick drain may be inserted and removed in two days. Drainage is a distinct disadvantage in these cases provided a clean operation can be performed. Chronic sinuses are likely to follow drainage, which greatly prolong convalescence. Even if the wound subsequently breaks down after complete closure the condition is not likely to be much worse than if drainage had been instituted at the time of operation. Wounds have been known to stay open three years, but this is unusual. In the cases of complete breakdown of the wound, secondary suture after the wound has cleaned up offers excellent results.

The severed ends of the ureter should be ligated and cauterized. The injection into the ureter of phenol, as has been advised, is unnecessary.

In cases which are advanced, or in which the capsule is densely adherent, or in which large pyonephritic lesions are present, subcapsular nephrectomy is extremely valuable and materially facilitates the operation and lessens the danger of hemorrhage. This operation is less satisfactory and more likely to be followed by wound infection than is the standard operation. It is, however, the operation of choice in certain types of cases in which operative difficulties are present that would materially increase the risk of an ordinary nephrectomy. Drainage should be instituted.

Watson and Cunningham (*loc. cit.*) have collected 201 cases of nephrectomy from the reports of Albarran, Krönelein, Israel, Kummel, and Rafin, in which the operative mortality was 5.8 per cent. Modern methods show an operative mortality of not over 1 to 3 per cent in the early cases and 10 to 15 per cent in the late ones. Among the 35 cases of renal tuberculosis operated upon in the Gynecological Service at the University Hospital there has been no operative mortality from any cause. Regarding the end results Walker (*Ann. Surg.*, 1907. 14:249, 388, 597) in a series of 210 patients showed 7 improved, 2 not improved and 15 temporarily improved and the remainder well. In 1912 Israel (*Cor.-Bl. f. schweiz, Aerzte.* Dec. 20, 1912) collected a series of 1023 nephrectomies from the literature. The mortality in the first six months was 13 per cent and as many more died later. About 65 per cent of cures may be expected and about 20 per cent more are improved. The prognosis is said to be somewhat more favorable in women than in men.

The degree of discomfort during convalescence due to vesical irritation is generally in direct ratio to the extent of involvement prior to operation. This tends to improve, but in some instances is a slow process and marked frequency and dysuria may continue for months.

Local applications are sometimes valuable. Generally there is a slow but progressive improvement and final clearing up. This course may be interrupted by attacks of ureteral colic simulating calculus especially in patients in whom there has been marked ureteritis. Tubercle bacillus and pus may continue in the urine for some time.

Nephrotomy may be of value as a palliative measure in cases in which collections of pus are present and in which nephrectomy is contraindicated. Occasionally nephrotomy may be employed as a preliminary to nephrectomy. Nephrotomy is rarely indicated. Resection of a part of the kidney is inadvisable. A few exceptional cases have been recorded which have been benefited by this operation. The fact that there is no known method by which the condition of the remaining portion of the kidney can be determined, coupled with the knowledge that in the majority of cases it is involved in the tuberculous process, makes this operation generally useless. In the ordinary case nephrectomy not only gives infinitely superior results but is associated with a shorter convalescence and a lesser operative mortality.

The question of operation in the presence of bilateral renal tuberculosis has recently attracted much attention. As a general rule nephrectomy in the presence of bilateral renal tuberculosis is contraindicated. It is recognized however that renal tuberculosis is often a slowly progressing lesion, and occasionally with what appears an advanced lesion on one side and an early one on the opposite, removal of the more diseased kidney may be a valuable palliative measure, and result in prolongation of life and temporary improvement. In the same type of case, especially if the more diseased kidney is the seat of a large pyonephritic collection, nephrotomy may be advisable.

Postoperative treatment after nephrectomy for renal tuberculosis is of the utmost importance, fresh air, nourishing diet, regular hours of sleep or, in general, the hygiene usually instituted for tuberculous patients, should be employed. It must not be lost sight of that these patients in addition to a long convalescence from a major operation are probably still the incumbents of a tuberculous ureteritis and cystitis, and also have a primary lesion often in the lung and must be treated accordingly. Urine analysis should be performed at regular intervals and the amount of urine passed should be carefully measured. The ingestion of moderately large quantities of water and a bland nonirritating diet is indicated. A warm equable climate is preferable. In the early and favorable cases in which there is little or no ureteral or vesical involvement, no local treatment is necessary. Frequently, however, in those cases which have suffered from vesical symptoms prior to operation there is a continuation of these, for a time at least, subsequent to operation. At times these symptoms are extremely distressing, and although there is nearly always an ultimate subsidence of the bladder symptoms, they may continue for weeks or even months. Under these circumstances in addition to the administration of large quantities of water and the elimination of irritant foods from the diet, the employment of urinary antiseptics is of value. In severe and long continued cases vesical irrigation with boric solution often gives relief. For the acute colicky attacks due to the ureter becoming more or less obstructed by pus or detritus nothing equals morphin by hypodermic and indeed it is the only thing that will give relief. Ureteral fistulae may develop and are especially likely in cases in which the drainage has been instituted and in which the ureter has been severed flush with the kidney.

Ordinary surgical cleanliness is sufficient in the majority of cases. If the condition persists the end of the ureter may be isolated, if necessary under anesthesia, and a few drops of phenol introduced through a ureteral catheter.

In nonoperative cases, palliative treatment consisting of hygiene, diet, etc., should be employed. Local treatment directed to the bladder is rarely productive of results. The injection into the bladder of two drams of a weak novocain solution gives temporary relief. Occasionally, where the bladder is markedly contracted forcible dilatation may effect an improvement. Marked relief sometimes follows the formation of a vesicovaginal fistula when the vesical pains and frequency are unbearable. It is important to make these patients as comfortable as possible. Opium or its derivatives are often indicated and are best administered per rectum or by hypodermic. There is danger of habit forming, but the cases are in any instance doomed and the suffering is often so extremely acute that the exhibition of morphin in large doses is the lesser of two evils. As has been stated, the tendency is to run a slow, progressive downward course with a duration of five to ten years.

# GYNECOLOGICAL AND OBSTETRICAL PATHOLOGY

ROBERT TILDEN FRANK, M.D.

## APPENDIX

Three years have elapsed since *Gynecological and Obstetrical Pathology* appeared. Much casuistic literature has accumulated, but this does not require extended mention in this appendix, nor does it warrant a full revision of the text. Two important advances will be referred to in some detail. The first deals with our increase in knowledge of the female sex cycle, the second refers to the entirely new aspect given to the subject of "chocolate cysts" of the ovary by Sampson's researches. Page references mentioned in square brackets will refer to the text of *Gynecological and Obstetrical Pathology*. No continuity could be maintained because of the variety of topics to be dealt with.

**Anatomy** [page 39].—Latarjet and Rochet (*Gynéc. et obst.* 1922. 6: 225) describe the pelvic ganglia, some situated on the lateral surfaces of the rectum, others on the sacro-uterine ligaments. Whitehouse and Featherstone (*Brit. M. J.* 1923. 2:406) have shown that the circular fibers of the uterus are stimulated by the sympathetic and inhibited by the lumbar cord, the reverse obtaining for the longitudinal fibers. Leveuf and Godard (*Rev. de chir.* 1923. 61:219) have studied the lymphatics of the uterus. Their plates are valuable.

[Page 70] A recent publication by Allen (*Am. J. Anat.* 1923. 31: 439) confirms the findings of Robinson (1918) in the ferret, showing that in the mouse also new "primitive" ova are formed from the germinal epithelium at each sex cycle by a process very analogous to spermatogenesis in the male. If these findings are applicable to all species, the belief that ova are direct descendants from the germ cells of the early embryo must be revised.

**Physiology** [page 74].—Long and Evans (*Mem. Univ. of Cal.*, "The Estrous Cycle in the Rat." 1922. 6) transplanted the ovaries of immature rats into mature castrates. When the grafts took the immature ovaries at once matured and functionated. This observation implies either a restraining influence in the immature subject, or the absence of some necessary factor before puberty.

[Page 82] My own observations and deductions enable me to-day (Frank. *Am. J. Obst. & Gynec.* 1924. 8:573) to simplify considerably the analysis of the physiology of the sex cycle. The growing follicle, as I stated in 1922 and before then [page 80], produces the premenstrual, or, using the more striking and adequate phrase, the *pregravid change* in the uterine mucosa. The mature follicle then ruptures and under proper conditions the ovum is impregnated in the tube. The time of ovulation being variable in the human species, follicle rupture may take place at any time from 1 to 25 days after cessation of the menses. The shell which harbored the ovulum continues the function of the granulosa, quickly changing to the corpus luteum, and maintains and accentuates the decidua in the uterus. The ovum then fixes in the prepared uterine mucous membrane. The placenta, as the corpus luteum becomes inactive, in turn takes up this protective and stimulating power over the uterus and breasts, producing the full hyperplasia necessary to harbor the rapidly growing ovum and to prepare the sex tract for parturition and successful lactation. This un-

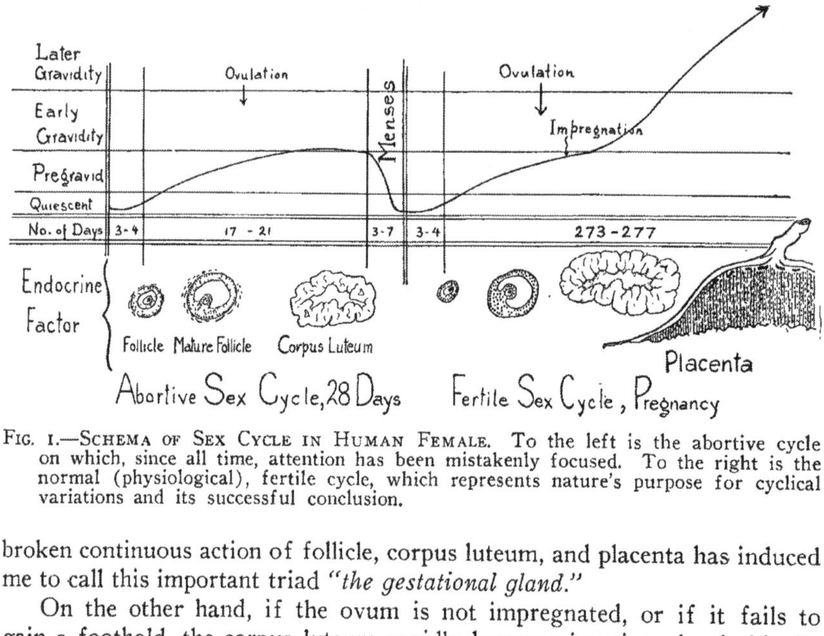


FIG. 1.—SCHEMA OF SEX CYCLE IN HUMAN FEMALE. To the left is the abortive cycle on which, since all time, attention has been mistakenly focused. To the right is the normal (physiological), fertile cycle, which represents nature's purpose for cyclical variations and its successful conclusion.

broken continuous action of follicle, corpus luteum, and placenta has induced me to call this important triad *"the gestational gland."*

On the other hand, if the ovum is not impregnated, or if it fails to gain a foothold, the corpus luteum rapidly becomes inactive, the decidually changed mucosa is suddenly deprived of its nutrition, necroses, and is cast off piecemeal (Schroeder. *Monatschr. f. Geburtsh. Gynaek.* 1914. 39:3; Lindner. *Ibid.* 1922. 57:119). The raw interior of the hyperemic uterus bleeds, thus producing the external signs of menstruation. In my opinion the older view that *menstruation corresponds to abortion of an unimpregnated ovum is fully justified.*

Almost all of the above changes can be artificially produced. By injecting follicle fluid into immature animals premature sex development can be obtained (Frank. 1922. *J. Am. M. Ass.* 1922. 78:181). Injection of follicle fluid or of its lipoid extract, into castrates (Frank. 1922, *vide ante;* Allen and Doisey. *J. Am. M. Ass.,* 1923. 81:819), as well as injection of corpus lutem or of placental lipoid extracts produce the preëstrual as well as estrual changes. (For literature see Frank. *Am. J. Obst. & Gynec.* 1924. 8:573, and Frank and Gustavson. *J. Am. M. Ass.* 1925. 84:1715.)

The breast changes taking place during each sex cycle in the human female have been described by Rosenburg (*Zentralbl. f. Gynäk.* 1923. 47: 111). These constant changes throw some light upon the frequent occurrence of mammary cancer in the female.

**Sterility** [page 82].—Mechanical interference with conception is now readily diagnosed by means of the Rubian insufflation test. Biological sterility due to a spermotoxin has been described by McCartney (*Am. J. Physiol.* 1923. 66:404). Reynolds and Macomber (*Fertility and Sterility in Human Marriage.* Saunders. 1924) ascribe importance to the diet, as well as to constitutional factors which lower the level of the threshold of reproduction. In other words, mechanical obstruction is now relegated to the background, while biological causes are emphasized. In my opinion chronic endocervicitis is still the most prolific source of "relative sterility."

**Vulva and Vagina** [page 107].—*Granuloma inguinale* appears to have existed endemically in the United States for some time but has only recently been recognized. A local papule develops on or near the genitals, breaks down and forms serpiginous, granulating, often nodular or warty lesions on the genitals, perineum, anus, suprapubic or inguinal regions. The fully developed lesions are elevated, bright red, bleed readily and, in the vagina, form doughy indurations. Microscopically warty areas and a non-specific granulomatous tissue is found. Deep scrapings may show capsulate bacteria (Donovan's organisms, calimatobacterium granulomatis, and spirochetes) but their etiological significance is uncertain. Antimony tartrate intravenously is specific. (For literature see Frank, *Southwestern Medicine,* Nov., 1923.)

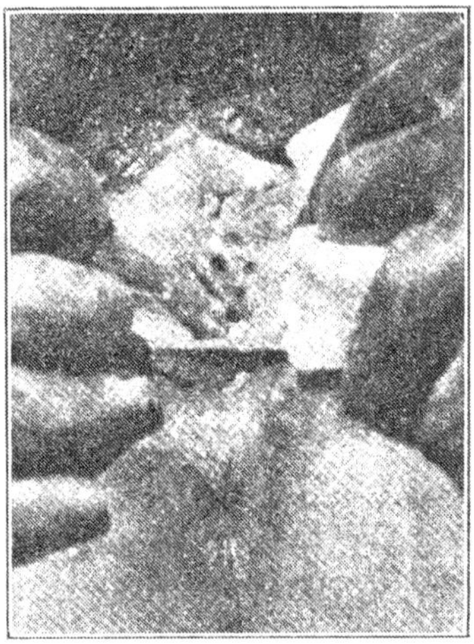

FIG. 2.—GRANULOMA INGUINALE IN A NEGRESS. Both labia minora and entrance of vagina involved. Velvety, bright strawberry-red lesions, bleeding readily, secreting a profuse, thin, fetid discharge. Vagina indurated where affected.

*Vulval and Vaginal Ulcers.*—Attempts to classify ulcers of this region have not been specially successful. Teague and Deibert (*J. of Urol.* 1920. 4: 543) have grown the organism of chancroid on clotted blood (see also *J. Med. Research.* 1922. 43: 61). In erosive vulvitis Driscoll (*Arch. f. Dermat. u. Syph.* 1920. 1:170) found a spirochete and vibrio. Aphthous, diphtheritic, dysenteric, and "veneroid" ulcers, the last looking like a mixed syphilitic and soft chancre, but self-limited (see Olson, *Arch f. Dermat. u. Syph.* 1920. 1:279) are described.

Under the title of "Ulcus vulvæ acutum," Lipschütz (*Dermatol. Studien, Unna und Rille.* Vol. 25. Voss. Leipzig. 1923) has written a monograph covering the subject of some of these indefinite ulcers. The lesions are not due to venereal causes, show a marked tendency to recurrence over periods of years, and appear in three forms—miliary, "veneroid," or gangrenous. From the ulcer the Bacillus crassus can be isolated. This bacillus is identical with the vaginal bacillus (lacticus) of Doederlein. The Doederlein bacillus according to Lipschütz may become pathogenic and is found in urethritis, endocervicitis, and even in salpingitis. The lesion is due to an inflammation of the capillaries and smallest venous radicals and characterized by a lymphocytic exudate into the tissues. My personal impression of this monograph is that it is not convincing.

[Page 148] *Tumors of the recto-vaginal septum* are rare. Herrmann (*Zentralbl. f. Gynäk.* 1922. 46: 1862) reported a lymphangio fibroma; Rivett (*Proc. Roy. Soc. Med.*, Sect. Obst. & Gynec. 1923. See *J. Obst. & Gynæc. Brit. Emp.* 1923. 30:485) described a calcified mass, while Szamek (*Zentralbl. f. Gynäk.* 1923. 47: 752) recorded a perivascular spindle cell sarcoma of this region.

**Malpositions, Prolapse** [page 165].—Traumatic displacement and prolapse of the uterus is certainly as uncommon as Mock implies (*J. Am. M. Ass.* 1922. 79:797). Unless infiltration of the pelvic floor is noted immediately after occurrence of the injury (hemorrhage), no evidence of medico-legal value is available.

Brettauer and Rubin (*Am. J. Obst. & Gynec.* 1923. 6: 696) have called attention to the fact that uncorrected uterine prolapse in 8 of 10 cases produced dilatation of one or both ureters due to constriction at the site of crossing of the uterine artery.

More and more attention is devoted to the observation that prolapse develops most often in individuals constitutionally handicapped by asthenia and infantilism (von Jaschke, *Arch. f. Gynæk.* 1923. 120:56).

**Uterus** [page 188].—*The cyclical changes* occurring in the uterine mucosa are now universally recognized and are but rarely mistaken for "endometritis." Schroeder and Neuendorff-Viek (*Arch. f. Gynæk.* 1921. 115: 15) show that acute endometrial infections do not affect the cyclical changes. Prolonged infections (which, I may add, are most unusual) reduce the development of the functional layer, until the final outcome may be the mucosa converted into an abscess lining (inert granulation tissue).

[Page 290] *Papilloma of the cervix*, a rare lesion, was omitted from my book. The accuminate condyloma is seen during pregnancy (usually in gonorrheal infection) and the true wart (not containing nevus cells) is a still rarer finding (Meyer, R. *Arch. f. Gynæk.* 1921. 115:167).

[Page 307] Systematic attempts to gage the degree of malignancy of corporeal cancer by its histology have been made by Mahle (*Surg., Gynec. & Obst.* 1923. 36: 385). He found that MacCarty's standard of cellular differentiation was an accurate guide in prognosis. Further confirmation is imperatively needed, for though the experience is universal, that "adenoma malignum" is the least malignant variety, it is less certain that the *clinical* degree of malignancy increases step by step with histological undifferentiation.

**Fallopian Tube** [page 329].—Successful cultivation of the gonococcus by reducing the oxygen tension has been described by Swartz, Shohl, and

Davis (*Johns Hopkins Hosp. Bull.* 1920. 31:449. No. 358). Kinsella, Broun, and Garcia (*J. Infect. Dis.* 1923. 32:1) stress the physical factors of the culture medium. Finally Torrey, Wilson, and Buckell (*Ibid.* 1922. 31:148) compare the discordant results of smears, cultures, and complement fixation. Our main reliance will still have to be placed upon the smear. It should be kept in mind that the Micrococcus catarrhalis cannot be differentiated from the gonococcus by morphological criteria (Shivers. *J. Am. M. Ass.* 1923. 80:1359).

**Ovary** [page 367].—*Transplantation of the ovaries* has never equaled the glowing expectations first entertained. Martin (*Surg., Gynec. & Obst.* 1922. 35:573) gives a full review of the literature. Autotransplantation offers some hope of success, homo- and heterotransplants offer none. DeBruyne (*Gynéc. et Obst.* 1922. 6:136) in 58 transplants after subtotal hysterectomy saw no signs of follicle ripening. The exception is supplied by Natrass (*Brit. M. J.* 1923, June 23. 1051) who nine and one half years after transplantation of both ovaries into the abdominal wall, the menstrual function being preserved, removed one graft and found normal graafian follicles, a corpus luteum and stroma.

[Page 385] Uterine bleeding often results from torsion of ovarian tumors, even before puberty and after the menopause. Moulonguet-Doléris (*Gynéc. et Obst.* 1924. 9:493) found that in one of every 4 ovarian growths bleeding occurred after the menopause without torsion of the pedicle. Of 7 uteri examined histologically 5 showed hyperplasia of the endometrium.

[Page 388] "The Life History of Ovarian Hematomas (Hemorrhagic Cysts) of Endometrial (Müllerian) Type," by John A. Sampson (*Am. J. Obst. & Gynec.* 1922. 4:451) has explained the origin of many hitherto puzzling "chocolate cysts" encountered in the pelvis. In 170 abdominal operations Sampson found 43 such cysts. According to the author uterine or tubal epithelium is extruded through the fallopian tube and is implanted in the ovary or on the pelvic peritoneum. The ovary acts as an incubator, small implants forming cysts, which become distended with menstrual blood and rupture, allowing secondary dissemination of the lining epithelium which then may show increased invasive power. Characteristic is the tarry (menstrual blood) content, the early tendency to rupture and to form dense adhesions (irritative peritonitis). If the epithelial lining is destroyed by pressure or by the menstrual reaction (?) the life of the cyst is self-terminated (Fig. 3). Where cellular stroma is encountered about the adenoma tubules Sampson derives the epithelium from the uterus; where cytogenic stroma is lacking he suggests a tubal origin. He considers these implantation-adenomas one of the main sources of ovarian cysts and carcinoma.

This paper is of great and fundamental importance. However, until further proof is offered I am still inclined to ascribe the origin of some adenomas to other causes [see page 213]. Moreover some of the minute "adenomas of the ovary" pictured by Sampson might well be interpreted as atypical follicle atresia. Experimental proof of the transplantability of endometrial tissue in the abdomen of the rabbit was presented by Jacobson (*Arch. Surg.* 1922. 5:281), clinical proof developed in a case of Lochrane's (*J. Obst. & Gynæc. Brit. Emp.* 1923. 30:213) in which an adenomyoma developed in the scar, four and one half years after ventrofixation, increasing with each menstruation.

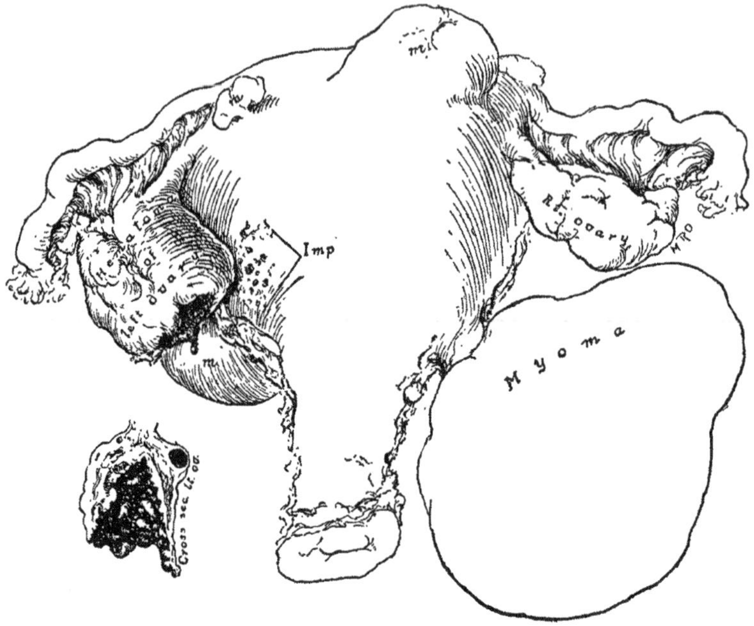


FIG. 3.—HEMATOMA OF ENDOMETRIAL TYPE OF THE LEFT OVARY, WITH PERFORATION; implantation adenoma (imp.) on the posterior surface of the uterus near the site of the perforation of the ovarian hematoma, multiple leiomyomas, early uterine pregnancy with typical decidual reaction of the lining of the ovarian hematoma, and the implantation adenoma of the posterior uterine wall. Posterior view of the specimen removed at operation (× 3/5). (From Sampson, *Am. J. Obst. and Gynec.,* 1922.)

**Obstetrics.**—The section in my book which dealt with obstetrics was of necessity much compressed. When a full revision is prepared the subject of "pregnancy and associated lesions" such as the effect of gestation on the special senses, on the circulatory system, on tuberculosis may well be considered. This applies as well to intercurrent diseases. To-day this would lead us too far afield.

Those interested in the causes of death in pregnancy, labor, and the puerperium can refer to the articles of Katz (*Arch. f. Gynaek.* 1921. 115:283) and Rosensohn (*Bull. Lying-in Hosp. N. Y.* 1923. 12:264).

Ovarian pregnancy has been observed so often that even the most skeptical must now be convinced of its occurrence. Convincing cases of primary abdominal pregnancy too have been observed (*Surg., Gynec.*

*& Obst.* 1921. 32:437, case II; Jacquin. *Gynéc. et Obst.* 1922. 5: 492) the ovum usually embedding near the bottom of the posterior culdesac.

Exception was taken to my statistics on tubal gestation [page 453], my material showing an excess of ruptures over tubal abortion (53: 31). Statistics vary widely with the type of gynecological service; Pollack, for example, in 307 cases found ruptured 31, tubal abortion 199, unruptured 39 (*Am. J. Obst. & Gynec.* 1921. 2:280). Mason and Storrs, on the other hand, reported 167 ruptures and only 75 abortions (*Boston M. & S. J.* 1923. 189: 914). The tube may resume normal function after the products of conception are removed as proved by the case of Barrows (see *Am. J. Obst. & Gynec.* 1921. 2: 567), in which only this tube remained and intra-uterine pregnancy took place two years later, and a similar one of Ramsay's (*Proc. Roy. Soc. Med.*, Sect. Obst. & Gynec. 1924. 17: 53).

[Page 457] In my book the subject of *premature separation of the normally situated placenta,* also called abruptio-placentae (Holmes) and uteroplacental apoplexy (Couvelaire), was inadvertently omitted. Concealed or external hemorrhage from this cause occurs more often than from placenta previa (about 1 in 200 pregnancies). Most cases are due to toxemia; a few may result from trauma. In severe cases the uterus resembles a huge ovarian cyst with twisted pedicle. Dark myometric and subperitoneal hemorrhages, most marked near the fundus and over the placental site, hemorrhages in the broad ligament and even in the adnexa, give the uterus a black-red, wet-leather appearance. Fissures through the peritoneal coat, in severe types account for the intraperitoneal accumulation of blood found. Microscopically an accumulation of fresh blood is found between the muscle bundles and even between individual muscle-fibers. The changes described in the decidua and uterine blood vessels are in no way pathognomonic. The placenta may show compression and indentation, if a retroplacental hematoma has formed. The condition is often fatal to the mother because the uterus has lost its contractility and death occurs from intra- and postpartum bleeding. The fetal mortality exceeds 90 per cent. An excellent résumé of the literature is given by Willson (*Surg., Gynec. & Obst.* 1922. 34:57; see also Scott. *Ibid.* 1924. 38: 450).

[Page 460] I am in full accord with Adair (*Tr. Am. Gynec. Soc.* 1923. 48: 190) who considers that *placental infarcts* are end products ascribable to many and varied causes. Chief among these he places endarteritis, periarteritis and thrombosis, localized hemorrhages due to static, traumatic, or toxic causes. Von Ravenstein (*Zentralbl. f. Gynäk.* 1923. 47: 727) could find no correspondence between infarcts and albuminuria. Talbot (*Surg., Gynec. & Obst.* 1921. 32: 552), without direct evidence, declares that infarcts "are a clinical record of the presence of bacteria in the blood stream of the pregnant woman." If this hypothesis were true, suppurative infarction would be of common occurrence, instead of the aseptic obliteration which is regularly found.

**Fetus.**—A separate chapter should be devoted to malformations and diseases of the fetus. At present it is not feasible to write this chapter. A few notes may prove of service.

Stratkosch (*Arch. f. Gynæk.* 1921. 115:408) has written a complete account of acardii.

Strachan (*Brit. M. J.* 1922. 2:80) describes maceration (non-syphilitic) as autolysis with edema of the interstitial tissue and extrusion of the red blood cells.

Capon (*J. Obst. & Gynæc. Brit. Emp.* 1922. 29:239) ascribes general edema of the fetus to obliteration of the intervillous space and polycythemia of the fetus.

Repeated malformations in succeeding pregnancies are discussed by Walther and Lelievre (*Bull. Soc. d'obst. & de gynéc. de Par.* 1923. 12:535), polycystic kidneys and meningocele recurring three times.

Fetal peritonitis is described by Westphal (*Monatschr. f. Geburtsh. u. Gynaek.* 1924. 66:245).

In these days of "operative midwifery" with version performed for almost any indication, Pierson's "Spinal and Cranial Injuries of the Baby in Breech Delivery" (*Surg., Gynec. & Obst.* 1923. 37:802) makes wholesome reading. Spinal cord hemorrhages, vertebral fractures, intracranial bleeding were found to be the causes of death.

Roentgen ray injury to the fetus is uncommon. Abels (*Wien. klin. Wchnschr.* 1924. 37:869) describes the birth of a small male with microcephaly and aplastic penis which he refers to x-raying of the uterus in the second and third month of pregnancy (?).

**Eclampsia** [page 486].—The statement in the original text that the necrotic areas in eclampsia are usually *central* was an error. The characteristic lesion is located in the *periphery* of the lobule. In spite of much casuistic and experimental work, no new light has been cast upon the causation of eclampsia. The latest detailed work is that of Hinselmann, *Die Eklampsie,* Fr. Cohen, Bonn, 1924.

**Internal Secretions** [page 499].—Hermaphroditism is really an endocrine disease, due to a bisexual anlage of the gonads. Consequent persistence of part or the whole of the müllerian and wolffian tubular system results. Young reports an interesting case (*Johns Hopkins Hosp. Bull.* 1924. 35:165) in which the psyche and secondary sex characters were male although the ovary functionated, the testis showing no spermatogenesis. An increasing number of cases like this, of true hermaphroditism, are being reported.

The most important new discovery in endocrinology and also in the entire field of medicine is the isolation of the active extract of the pancreas by Banting, Best, and others. (For original article see *Canad. M. Ass. J.* 1922. 12:141.)

Insulin has proved a boon, enabling us to control serious diabetes, and rapidly to overcome ketosis. A huge literature dealing with insulin has already accumulated.

Abel has isolated a tartrate of the pituitary extract but has been unable to determine the composition of the active principle.

Researches on the female sex hormone show that the active fraction follows lipoid extractives, that the active principle may be obtained free of phosphorus, nitrogen or cholesterol (Frank. *Am. J. Obst. & Gynec.* 1924. 8:573), and that the vaginal smear method of Long and Evans. ("The Estrous Cycle in the Rat," *Mem. Univ. of Cal.* 1922. Vol. VI) furnishes an easy and reliable qualitative test of potency on the living rat, the animal being avalaible for repeated tests. (Allen and Doisey. *J. Am. M. Ass.* 1923. 81:819.)

Most of the enormous literature of endocrinology is so largely clinical that no further discussion is indicated here.

# BIRTH INJURIES OF THE CHILD

HUGO EHRENFEST, M.D.

## APPENDIX

A search through recent medical literature for contributions to the problem of the traumatization of the child in birth carries conviction that serious concern with this question to-day is widespread among all the special branches of medical practice.

Approximately two hundred papers have been published within the past three years alone which deal with various injuries of this kind and with their effect on the physical and mental development of children surviving such injuries. Many of these contributions markedly augment information at present available concerning the pathology and etiology of these lesions. A few more of well-known pathologic conditions and clinical entities, still designated as congenital to indicate their intra-uterine and developmental origin, now have been definitely placed into the group of intranatal injuries.

More extensively than heretofore pathologists and neurologists, as well as surgeons, laryngo-otologists, and ophthalmologists have participated in the discussion of this complex question which in the main claims primarily the interest of obstetricians and pediatricians.

As might be expected, the bulk of these newer contributions considers injuries to the central nervous system and their sequelæ, the most frequent and, at the same time, the gravest type of traumatization of the newborn.

**Intracranial Injuries.**—It seems that it now is accepted as an established fact that approximately one-half of all infants, either stillborn or dying within the first few days of life, reveal at autopsy some sort of laceration of the dura mater, or more particularly of the tentorium. Thus, in one of the largest number of observations more recently summarized, Holland found tears in the dura mater in 81 of 167 fetuses, and in 64 of them he discovered a bilateral laceration of the tentorium, none of these lacerations being necessarily responsible for the infant's death. Lower figures, as those given by Keene, strongly suggest a not quite perfect postmortem technic.

Recent investigations agree with the claim, made some time ago by German writers, that only approximately one-half of these lacerations cause sufficient hemorrhage to account satisfactorily for the death. In the other half, then, they merely express the potential risk to the infant in case such a laceration accidentally were to have involved a larger vessel, and furthermore demonstrate the ever present danger to the integrity of the dura from external mechanical factors.

The problem of intracranial stress as the result of changes in the shape of the skull during the process of moulding is most lucidly presented by Holland. He supports the opinion of former investigators that compression of the head raises the vault of the cranium and with it the falx, causing the falx itself or the tentoria to tear when overstretched. It is the inevitable, exaggerated compression of the skull in face and brow presentations, and its rapid compression in the delivery of the aftercoming head in breech labors, which account for the high percentage of lacerations and hemorrhages among infants born in this manner.

With certain features of this theory Greenwood takes issue. He made plaster-of-Paris casts of the newborn's head, reaching from below the frontal eminences to below the occiput, including thus the whole of the skull surface subjected to moulding. Another similar cast was taken a week or so later. These casts permit very exact measurements in various directions, and conclusions drawn from them force us to modify some of our ideas concerning the changes of configuration resulting from moulding.

These exact studies leave no doubt that in normal cases of vertex presentations the passage of the suboccipitobregmatic circumference through the pelvic brim does not, as now assumed, increase the vertical diameter of the cranium. On the contrary, the tendency is to shorten this diameter and to cause merely an overlapping of the two parietal bones. The lengthening of the head is anteroposterior and not vertical. That in many vertex cases dural septa are torn is an admitted fact, but at least in normal vertex presentations this injury cannot be explained by any raising of the cranial vault. This mechanism, however, undoubtedly might be responsible for dural lacerations in occipitoposterior presentations, in which there usually is some deflexion; in brow presentations, and especially in breech labors. In the aftercoming head, as can be clearly shown, the vertical diameter always becomes increased. This lengthening begins with the very first contact of the head with the pelvic brim and, if there is any difficulty, the elongation will be extreme and beyond compatibility with life.

Greenwood is convinced that the Schultze method of resuscitation might be responsible for dural injuries in some cases, as is also claimed by Siegmund.

Beitzke thinks that the direction of the compression, occipitofrontal or bilateral, determines whether the tentorium is torn approximately in the middle of its free edge or at the site of its attachment to the falx. The former type of lesion is more likely to occur during excessive bilateral compression because it also causes the cerebellum to be pushed upward against the tentorium, a point already emphasized by Wilke in 1912.

By far the most significant result of recent studies consists in new information concerning the character and the later consequences of apparently common lesions of the brain substance sustained during labor. This work, chiefly done in the Pathologic Institute at Frankfort by Philip Schwartz and his coworkers, is presented by Schwartz in an exhaustive, well-illustrated and most instructive monograph of two hundred pages and more briefly summarized by Fischer and Siegmund.

One can readily agree with the allegation that the almost general adoption of Beneke's method for the study of intracranial pathology of the newborn rather one-sidedly brought about an overestimate of the significance of dural lesions, and inevitably caused the now evident neglect of injuries to the brain substance itself.

If the skull is opened by a method very similar to the customary technic in the adult, but with the skull flaps made larger (by running the incision anteriorly lower down to the orbital ridge, laterally down to the attachment of the ear, and posteriorly below the transverse sinus) it is possible, while removing the hemispheres in toto, to inspect first the tentorium and then the falx. After a preliminary hardening in formalin solution, Schwartz studied the brain histologically. Hemorrhages or distinct areas of degeneration in the substance of the brain, outside the known and fairly common pial and tentorial hemorrhages, can even macroscopically be recognized in 65 per cent of all infants up to the age of five months. Their arrangement and localization can leave no doubt concerning their origin. Their distribution clearly expresses traumatization of the brain by the mechanism of labor.

The hemorrhages are within the area of the branches of the vena magna Galeni, vena terminalis, vena lateralis ventriculi, ramus ventricularis of the vena basalis, and vena chorioidea. The areas of soft degeneration lie chiefly in the white substance of the hemispheres and in regions drained by the vena terminalis and the vena lateralis ventriculi. Often extensive areas of the nucleus caudatus are found destroyed by hemorrhages from the vena terminalis.

As clearly demonstrated by Schwartz, the actual histopathologic condition in each individual observation stands in a very definite relation to the duration of extra-uterine life. It is Schwartz's belief that the entire problem can be understood fully only by extending such exact histologic investigations to all infants dying up to 30 days after birth and even later. Thus he arrived at the conclusion that there are but a few infants that fail to reveal at least some traces of such traumatic brain lesions.

There unquestionably exists a typical progression of histologic changes, leading from hematoma through necrosis or fatty degeneration of the glia, to diffuse sclerosis, cyst formation, porencephaly, etc. In the belief of Siegmund the entire further development of the infant's brain to a great extent is determined by disturbances set up by birth, an opinion similarly but more emphatically expressed by Ylppoe, who asserts that intracranial traumatic lesions, by him discovered in 90 per cent of all prematurely born infants, actually determine whether they will live and how they will later develop.

Fischer summarizes the findings, presented in all their details in Schwartz's monograph, as follows:

Hemorrhages in the brain substance occur in the newborn chiefly in two forms: (1) Very small, and occasionally larger, isolated hematomas in the white substance, radiating in an almost typical manner from the walls of the two lateral ventricles; (2) a very typical complex of hemorrhages, arranged strandlike, often in both hemispheres, distinctly ascribable to an injury of the vena terminalis, a type first described by Schwartz and since confirmed by others.

Outside these hemorrhages there can be seen opaque, grayish yellow spots, usually in the immediate neighborhood of the lateral ventricles, which under the microscope are found to be anemic, necrotic areas, or fields showing a softening from fatty degeneration.

The dependence at least of the hemorrhages upon birth trauma seemed evident from the start but very careful investigations finally established as well the relation of the necrotic or fatty degenerated areas to this trauma. If the degeneration is diffuse its gradual development into porencephaly can be demonstrated.

That the skull represents the all-important protective factor was convincingly shown by control studies made on the brain of newborn animals (calves, dogs, and cats) with thick bones and no fontanels. In not a single instance could such anomalies be discovered in the brain of these animals. Furthermore, in the newborn infants, traumatization of this character invariably was found more often and more extensively in the prematurely born and in infants with soft skull bones.

Direct pressure, strong compression of the entire brain, shearing, and a sort of concussion of the brain are the traumatizing factors. They are assumed by these authors to cause circulatory disturbances through their effect on the vasomotor nervous system. Either stasis or anemia is the primary result which then apparently forms the causative factors for the structural changes.

Fischer believes that Schwartz's original theory is correct, namely, a suction effect is created on the part of the head exposed within the area of the dilated cervix by the difference between the higher intrauterine and the lower outer atmospheric pressure.

It seemed natural that both the immediate and the early symptoms of such traumatization of the brain should resemble those of a concussion of the brain. As a matter of fact much clinical evidence now has been adduced to support strongly such a view.

Stern and Schwartz examined one hundred live newborn babies up to the age of 10 days and found in most of them periods of nystagmus alternating with intervals during which this anomaly could not be seen. Most often the nystagmus started spontaneously, in other cases the movements could be brought on simply by a slight turn of the head to one side. The horizontal type of nystagmus predominated, and only in four babies was the vertical type present.

This rhythmic rolling of the eyeballs was most marked within the first few hours after delivery. The older the child became, the smaller were the excursions, the longer the intervals between the attacks of nystagmus. Of 44 infants, in whom all the conditions of labor were perfectly normal, 15 had no nystagmus, while of 11 babies, born in abnormal presentations, all showed the anomaly. Out of 24 cases of contracted pelvis, 20 had a spontaneous nystagmus, and in three of the remaining four instances without nystagmus, the pelvic deformity was very slight. Of 38 first-born children only 8 failed to exhibit the anomaly, while of 52 babies of multiparous mothers 13 had no nystagmus. These same authors were able to demonstrate convincingly the relation both of frequency and duration of nystagmus to the degree of moulding of the head and as well as to the duration of the second stage of labor. One might well accept their conclusion that the dependence of nystagmus upon some traumatization of the brain in birth now can be considered as established.

Berberich and Wieders assumed that mechanical influences capable of affecting the brain to such an extent could not fail to exert some deleterious effect also on other organs of the head. Stump, Sicherer, and more recently Jacobs, have proved the high incidence of retinal hemorrhages in newborn infants as the expression of a birth trauma of some sort. Berberich and Wieders also investigated spontaneous and experimental nystagmus of the infant by employing both the caloric test and the turning table. The overwhelming majority of infants with deficient caloric reaction they found to be spasmophilics, idiots, epileptics, or neuropathics. The turning table gave results which in general exactly coincided with the caloric tests. All their findings strongly support the assumption of a serious traumatization of the brain.

Distinct alterations of the inner ear, including hemorrhages, have been discovered in the newborn by Voss.

Schwartz feels that the almost physiologically positive Babinski reflex of the newborn, recently found positive in 43 per cent of 88 normal and healthy infants within the first week of life by De Angelis, will have to be studied and analyzed in the light of all this newer information concerning the condition of the brain immediately after birth. He doubts that this inverted plantar reflex has anything to do with impairment or underdevelopment of the pyramids but believes it more likely dependent upon an injury of the corpus striatum.

Observations of peculiar attacks of arrest of breathing in newborn and young infants, a state of normal respiration suddenly and repeatedly interrupted by periods of apnea and cyanosis, have occasionally been recorded in pediatric literature. Recently, Still dealt with this perplexing condition and expressed the belief that these attacks must be due to some affection of the respiratory center itself. A most substantial basis has been furnished for this theory by Kirkwood and Meyers in a thorough study of a case of inspiratory apnea ending fatally. This infant appeared to be normal and well on the first day and did not manifest the first signs of trouble until the third day. It suddenly ceased to breathe for a short while and turned blue, then again breathed normally. Several similar attacks recurred. During the state of apnea some slight twitching was noted; a turning of the eyes, etc., and later convulsions appeared and the baby suddenly died.

Lundsden, who recently had made extensive investigations on cats concerning the exact location of the automatic respiratory center, performed the autopsy on this infant. He discovered hemorrhages in the pons which, in his opinion, paralyzed this center and therefore Kirkwood and Meyers suggest, with seeming justification, that minute hemorrhages in the pons probably are not infrequent in the newborn and might occasionally represent the not recognized cause of a neonatal death.

Behrendt emphasized the fact that "persistent spitters" among very young infants often show various symptoms of nervous hypersensitiveness, are spasmophilic or have tremors. This identical observation was recorded by Dollinger and, since among his own cases many of these babies have been born after difficult labors. he concludes that the evident hypersensitiveness, presumably in part expressed in this habitual vomiting, might be ascribed to the traumatization of the brain in birth. This explanation appeals to Schwartz who, like Ylppoe, is surprised that obstetricians and pediatricians so long have been satisfied in applying to definite clinical pathological conditions such terms as asphyxia, debility, atrophy, or spasmophilia, which in the adult never express anything but a mere symptom. He feels that his own investigations at least justify the hope that all these conditions some day possibly will be brought into a direct and specific relation to certain brain lesions sustained in birth. Foerster's recent studies concerning the athetotic striatum syndrome seem suggestive to Schwartz, but he objects to their classification as congenital, since more intensive study of the corpus striatum in the newborn might yet establish the intranatal origin of this syndrome.

When Kirby, in a careful analysis of all available information concerning congenital oculofacial paralysis, arrives at the final conclusion that no really satisfactory explanation for the occurrence of this condition is extant, the thought must suggest itself that here also we possibly deal only with the sequela of an intracranial birth injury—a possibility not even considered by him.

The complexity of the diversified lesions within and on the surface of the brain, produced by the traumatism of moulding, their usual multiplicity, peculiar distribution and wide variation as to size of the resulting hematoma, all these many factors explain why it is impossible to evolve a definite picture of the symptomatology of intracranial birth hemorrhages; why in the greatest majority of instances the lesion cannot be satisfactorily localized even when certain clinical manifestations or findings establish its existence. Cameron, Capon, Henkel, Holland, and others deal with the early general symptomatology which by now is well known: anomalies of respiration, cyanosis, inability to suckle, twitching, convulsions, paralysis, bulging of fontanels, separation of sutures, etc., but they are unable to offer any new helpful suggestions in regard to better evaluation and interpretation of such findings.

The long appreciated value of a spinal puncture for the diagnosis of intracephalic hemorrhage is emphasized or, as I would say, overemphasized by Sharpe in several papers. The mere presence of blood in the spinal puncture fluid can hardly be accepted as proof positive of an intracranial hemorrhage, and a recognized authority on spinal fluid, Levinson, quite recently wrote: "Obtaining bloody fluid is possibly the most frequent mishap in spinal puncture. It happens to both the inexperienced and the experienced. The blood is due to injury produced to the plexus of veins in the canal."

It furthermore might be doubted that a seemingly increased pressure of the spinal fluid, ascertained at the time of puncture, is of any great value for the diagnosis of increased intracranial pressure due to hemorrhage. It so happens that I discussed this very point with Professor Baranyi and he assured me, as have other experienced pediatricians, that the outcome of the measurement of this pressure is so greatly dependent upon the position of the baby at the time of the puncture, upon the character of respiration, and is so markedly influenced by crying, that the actual figures obtained in this manner are practically void of any significance.

The problem of immediate diagnosis is further complicated by the fact that symptoms, even of evident hemorrhage, may not appear until much later. A somewhat extreme but most instructive observation of this sort is recorded by Schele. This baby died rather unexpectedly when six weeks old. Autopsy showed a large subdural hemorrhage from a deep tentorial tear. Since this baby, to Schele's best knowledge, had not sustained a head trauma since birth, he assumed that a small tear, occurring at birth, did not heal properly, possibly as the result of an intercurrent acute febrile condition, and later reopened and further extended into the sinus transversus.

The delayed appearance of the signs of hemorrhage in some cases undoubtedly is due to persistence of a slight hemorrhage from a small vessel on account of the inability of the blood to coagulate properly. However, it is not justifiable to claim, as recently done by Kaiser, that a hemorrhagic diathesis often is the direct and sole cause of an intracephalic hemorrhage of the newborn. I take issue with Munro and Eustis for classifying hemorrhagic diathesis as one of the immediate etiologic factors in their grouping of the causes of cranial hemorrhages, and Conkey also feels that at present the hemorrhagic disease theory is overstressed to the exclusion of the causative mechanical and traumatic factors. It is true that Cruickshank, in his report of an analysis of the pathologic findings in 400 newborn infants, assigns first place to hemorrhagic disease as the chief cause of hemorrhages, but it should not be overlooked by writers quoting him that he speaks of all types of hemorrhages in the various tissues and organs of the newborn infant.

In my belief, the primarily traumatic origin of intracranial birth lesions now has been definitely established by the comparative studies of Schwartz on the brains of newborn infants and of newborn animals with hard skulls and no fontanels, mentioned in foregoing pages, and furthermore is convincingly demonstrated by all recent information concerning the high frequency of such injuries in breech labors, as well as in prematurely born infants.

Cruickshank offers the following figures: In 47 per cent of mature and 52 per cent of premature infants, in whom a tentorial tear was discovered at necropsy, a breech delivery had taken place. Of 81 infants with dural injuries, reported in Holland's series of 167 fetuses, 35 were either breech or version cases. In another paper Holland states that tentorial tears occur in 88 per cent of dead fetuses after breech labors, a figure given also by Crothers. In Saenger's belief no mechanism of labor is as dangerous to the child as the delivery of the aftercoming head. Of 23 children delivered in this manner, who came to autopsy, only three failed to show tentorial tears.

This high incidence of fatal intracranial lesions in breech labors can be plausibly explained only by decidedly unfavorable, mechanical factors inherent to the abnormal mechanism in the delivery of the head (Capon, Crothers, Greenwood, Saenger), though admittedly the risk is increased by undue haste during extraction of the head as emphasized by Holland, Pierson, myself, and others.

The immediate dependence of intracranial injuries upon birth trauma, however, probably is yet more convincingly shown by the fact that the ratio of their frequency and particularly the degree of their seriousness are directly proportionate to the stage of prematurity. Beyond question the skull bones represent the protective factor of greatest importance. Hard-skulled full term infants are less exposed to the damage of excessive external trauma and of exaggerated moulding. This latter fact was well illustrated in one of my cases.

The shape of the soft and elastic cranium of the premature infant is easily and often quickly altered to a dangerous and disastrous degree. The obstetrician must never forget that this exaggerated configuration, as definitely established by careful observations, can be effected also by the soft portions of the birth channel (Vogel), by a not completely dilated cervix, a rigid perineum, or a narrow vulval ring. This accident is particularly prone to occur when fast expulsion takes place, that is, in labors which, to the satisfaction of the mother, are easy and quick.

Raisz discovered in 81 autopsies of full term newborns, exactly as in the 42 autopsies of premature infants, signs of intracranial hemorrhage in 33.3 per cent; when he, however, considered the number of instances in which such a hemorrhage actually was responsible for death, he found among the full term infants fatal hemorrhages only in 5.12 per cent, but in 23.8 per cent of the premature infants.

Possibly of some significance for our problem is the recent observation of Reis that the greatest increase in the blood-pressure of newborn babies can be ascertained in those delivered by means of a midplane forceps or version extraction, with a lesser degree of elevation after the application of only a low forceps. He concludes that this increase of blood-pressure seemingly is due to an increased traumatization of the head. Though this rise in blood-pressure is not strikingly large, it might, in my opinion, present some factor in the causation of hemorrhages and particularly in premature babies.

A factor of great weight, however, is the evident fragility of the blood vessels in premature infants. Two newer contributions of Ylppoe must be mentioned in this connection. Hemorrhages of various kinds represent a characteristic difference in the clinical pathology of the young infant as compared with the adult. Ylppoe experimentally produced skin hemorrhages by creating a negative pressure by means of a suction bulb. In this manner he ascertained that in infants, weighing less than 1000 Gms., a pressure of 150 mm. Hg is sufficient to cause hemorrhage owing to the rupture of vessels. At a weight between 2000 and 2500 Gms. the required pressure was 400 mm. Hg, while in infants of 3000 Gms. and above, this pressure had to be raised to 520 mm. Hg to cause hemorrhage. These findings, at least in part, would explain hemorrhages in the premature infant, if we take into consideration the fact that the average of normal pressure in delivery at 250 mm. Hg for small premature infants actually transgresses the resistance of their blood vessels. This theoretical deduction he was able to establish as correct in another series of observations in which he demonstrated an inverse ratio of the frequency of brain hemorrhages to the degree of development. He found brain hemorrhages in 90 per cent of infants weighing less than 1000 gms., in 76.5 per cent weighing between 1000 and 1500 Gms., in 35.3 per cent of those between 1500 and 2000 Gms., and in 26.7 per cent weighing between 2000 and 2500 Gms. He feels certain that the further development of a premature infant is actually determined in the main by two factors, by its birth weight and by the degree of its traumatization in birth. Among premature infants, later in life, appear with striking frequency pathologic conditions, which are clearly referable to the central nervous system, and especially anomalies of intelligence.

In a large series of premature babies which he was able to follow for a longer time there were 7 to 8 per cent of imbeciles and idiots, 3 per cent alone developed a typical Little disease. He calculates that 40 per cent of premature infants, which had supposedly spasmophilic convulsions in the first and second year of life, later manifested evidences of cerebral defects of varying degrees, very often expressed as deficiency of mentality.

This problem of the relation of meningeal birth hemorrhages to later faulty physical and mental development, outside of Schwartz and others already quoted, is thoroughly discussed also by Cameron and Osman, Gordon, Hamill, and others. Stroehm, Ceelen, Schwartz, and Siegmund deny the existence of an encephalitis interstitialis of young infants as first described by Virchow. Burhans and Gerstenberger confirm the assertion of Rosenberg or Finkelstein that an internal hemorrhagic pachymeningitis in early infancy is more common than is generally believed. They feel certain that in some infants a subacute pachymeningitis originally resulting from a birth hemorrhage, later is rendered acute by some further physical injury.

An interesting historical outline of gradual change in views concerning the significance of convulsions in early life to later epilepsy can be found in an article by Patrick and Levy. In their own studies they were able to ascertain for 500 cases of idiopathic epilepsy an incidence of early convulsions amounting to probably more than 20 per cent, while in another group of 752 unselected infants and children the frequency of early convulsions amounted only to about 4.2 per cent, about one-fifth that of the epileptic group. Thus they are forced to conclude that the presence of an infantile convulsion *per se* multiplies the individual's ordinary chances for later epilepsy at least by five. However, there is a preponderating number of but one single infantile convulsion in the non-epileptic group.

A careful analysis of the figures presented by these writers reveals still another fact, seemingly important to the obstetrician though not stressed by them. In the epileptic group I find the incidence of convulsions to be almost twice as large within the first four weeks postpartum, and three times as large within the first five months of life, than in the corresponding ages of the non-epileptic group. If we admit that birth trauma plays a part in the causation of early convulsions, the conclusion strongly suggests itself from these figures that it also might be an etiological factor of some importance in the occurrence of epilepsy.

No truly new suggestions have been offered of late concerning the treatment of cerebral hemorrhages of the newborn. As far as simplicity and usefulness are concerned, lumbar puncture, repeated if necessary several times, remains in the forefront. This procedure is most enthusiastically supported, especially by Sharpe. Brady, who several years ago strongly advocated this simple and fairly safe operation, in a recent paper details a case in which he performed with perfect success a puncture of the cisterna magna. In his opinion this high puncture should be done whenever, in the presence of an evident hemorrhage, the customary spinal puncture fails to withdraw blood. In this manner it might be possible to save babies who heretofore have been lost owing to dry taps on lumbar puncture. His own case probably is the first one on record of seemingly complete recovery after a cisternal puncture for cerebral hemorrhage.

Ballance and Ballance advocate prompt operation in all cases of skull fracture "not only to obviate impending death but as well, in case of recovery, to anticipate and prevent paralysis, amentia, or epilepsy." It is their belief that infants bear these operations well if they are carried out with greatest gentleness and with every effort to prevent the loss of blood.

Of special interest to the obstetrician necessarily prove recent contributions dealing with the problem of prevention of intracranial damage in birth.

At present the view prevails that the main factor in the causation of tears in the dural septa is the trauma of exaggerated or rapid compression of the fetal head. Of only secondary, though admittedly considerable, importance in the origin of hemorrhages are: Distension of blood-vessels or sinuses owing to asphyxia; the fragility of the vessel walls in the premature infant, and a hemorrhagic diathesis which favors the gradual escape of a large quantity of blood even from small vessels. More recently, and chiefly through the work of Schwartz, multiple hemorrhages and degenerative processes within the brain substance have been brought into immediate etiologic relation to certain circulatory changes, hyperemia or anemia, both the result either of vasomotor disturbances or of an uneven blood distribution, due to the suction effect exerted by the lower outer atmospheric pressure on the portion of the head exposed within the area of the dilated cervix.

A clear conception of all these various causative factors enables us to develop certain rules for an effective prophylaxis.

We should not make use of an artificial method of delivery which tends to increase further an already existing cranial stress in a certain direction. This point is very lucidly set forth in the paper of Greenwood already mentioned: "Forceps will increase the danger to the child if it increases compression of an already compressed diameter. Forceps may be to the good, if it compresses a diameter compensatorily lengthened by the moulding, thus actually affording relief of tension on the septa." Theoretically, at least, it then would seem reasonable that the application of the forceps in a direction approaching the anteroposterior diameters of the head would imply not only less risk but might be a means of reducing the anteroposterior strain. On the other hand, from this same viewpoint, forceps would seem especially risky in brow and occipitoposterior presentations, and also on the aftercoming head, because under these conditions the forceps very likely would tend to increase further the already present vertical elongation of the cranium, which proves so particularly dangerous to the tentorium. Therefore, no means should be spared in the effort to obtain better flexion of the partially extended head, to change an occipitoposterior into an anterior presentation, or to obviate a breech labor by external version.

The particular usefulness of the Kielland forceps for rotating the head is emphasized by Saenger, who failed to discover an intra-cranial hemorrhage in any of his own cases where this forceps alone had been employed. However, it is not surprising that such hemorrhages also have been recorded after the use of the Kielland forceps since as a matter of fact they do occur after spontaneous labors of women with perfectly normal pelves.

The stress, due to vertical elevation of the cranium of the aftercoming head during a breech delivery, is relieved by pressure on the head from above which not only reduces required traction from below but also produces and maintains better flexion of the head. This latter important effect, in my belief, too often is not sufficiently appreciated. Appropriate help on the part of the assistant, who exerts this suprapubic pressure, implies the necessity that the direction of this pressure be not straight downward but always oblique, either from the left or the right according to the position of the occiput. This suprapubic force, especially during a uterine contraction, or when combined with traction from below, as shown by Crothers, must not be too strong, since otherwise collapse or death of the infant might result from the resulting herniation of the medulla through the foramen magnum.

The acknowledged etiologic significance of an anomaly in the coagulability of the fetal blood is fully taken into account in the practice, probably to-day a routine in most obstetric clinics, of giving to every infant which exhibits symptoms even only suggestive of hemorrhage, prophylactically a subcutaneous injection of from 10 to 30 c.c. of the father's or mother's blood. Falls prefers citrated blood injected into the jugular vein.

The evident vulnerability of the blood vessels in the premature infant makes it necessary to refrain from all medication or operative measures which hasten the passage of the child through not fully dilated soft portions of the birth canal.

More perplexing from the standpoint of prevention prove the risks inherent in unequal distribution of the blood within sinuses and vessels, expressing itself in either localized anemia or congestion. This latter condition obviously also is closely connected with general asphyxiation of the fetus, another element in the causation of hemorrhages. Must we try to overcome seemingly excessive or long-continued compression of the head by a forceps extraction as soon or even before we notice certain symptoms which supposedly indicate beginning asphyxiation? Gamper reminds us that to-day every obstetrician very naturally will endeavor to find the answer to the question: Is intracranial damage more often the result of failure to use forceps at the proper time or the direct result of their application?

Personally I have come to the conclusion that a definite answer to this question never can be formulated. In the light of our present knowledge concerning late effects of cranial birth lesions it is entirely illogical to gauge the risk of the forceps extraction or of any other obstetrical operation solely by fetal mortality statistics. Furthermore, the specific restriction of the application of the forceps at "the proper time," neither too early nor too late, actually is void of any real meaning, because it leaves the decision as to the propriety of the time unavoidably to the judgment of the operator. That this judgment, even among recognized experts, varies within very wide limits is clearly seen in the statistics from different large obstetric clinics. A calculation of the danger of forceps extraction from such really incomparable statistics carries no conviction, as pointed out by Gamper. If one simply compares the forceps frequency of a certain clinic with its neonatal mortality, support is found for the view of Heinlein that in general there probably exists an optimum of forceps frequency which lies between 2 and 3 per cent of all deliveries. It seems that a higher rate of forceps application often is associated with a higher fetal mortality. But, on the other hand, a well-marked conservatism does not necessarily cause immediate harm, in my opinion, as demonstrated by figures from the Frauenklinik in Graz, presented by Santner: In a total of 21,140 deliveries, forceps were applied in only 0.82 per cent of the cases with a total fetal mortality of 2.37 per cent, which as shown by Santner is a lower mortality than in any other reported large series with higher forceps incidence. "We believe," he writes, "that careful preservation of physiologic and normal action of the natural forces results in the best and safest form of delivery. If they seem insufficient we first try to strengthen and support them, and only if we fail in this endeavor, or if other threatening signs force interference, only then we resort to instruments or other artificial means."

No one familiar with the problem of cranial traumatization in birth can fail to agree heartily with this sound conclusion and advice. Of course, this does not mean that one should unconcernedly watch a head pressing hour after hour through the pelvic outlet against an unyielding perineum since "this is inviting disaster" as Greenwood very appropriately states. In such a situation the proper treatment consists in episiotomy, and if then expulsion does not follow, in gentle extraction with the forceps.

It can never be justifiable to apply forceps simply for the purpose of shortening labor in the interest of the mother. Even the mere changing of the fetal heart rate offers no indisputable indication for immediate interference.

It seems generally accepted, Frey points out, that a slowing of fetal heart sounds below 100 during two or three succeeding intervals between contractions is the sign of fetal asphyxiation. Since the pressure of the contracting uterine wall undeniably must be a factor in the causation of this asphyxia it is only reasonable, if immediate delivery is not feasible, to relieve this pressure temporarily by the administration of narcotics, a suggestion made some time ago by Seitz. Frey prepared a patient for forceps extraction because the fetal heart had slowed down to a seemingly dangerous degree. With the patient in deep anesthesia he realized that delivery at that moment was not possible. Several hours later the patient expelled spontaneously a perfectly fresh, not asphyxiated child. This observation induced him to experiment with the systematic use of chloroform for the purpose of overcoming threatened intrauterine asphyxiation of the fetus. From observations made on 35 cases he concludes that chloroform is indicated if the fetal heart rate remains below 100 for the entire interval between two contractions. If within the next ten to fifteen minutes, with the patient kept under anesthesia, the fetal pulse returns approximately to normal, the administration of the anesthetic can be stopped. Only if the fetal pulse in this time does not slacken considerably the justification for operation is given.

The practical importance of this novel suggestion is shown by the fact that in deliveries, both at home and in hospitals, the assumption of fetal asphyxiation leads to about 70 per cent of all artificial deliveries.

A slowing of heart beats in the second stage of labor, states Bartram, might mean an accumulation of carbon dioxid. The interference with the required oxygen supply to the fetus might be due to abnormal conditions either in the placenta or in cord circulation, or indicate as well an existing intracranial hypertension. If the hypertension is caused by an intracranial hemorrhage, operative delivery obviously will fail to bring help; if due solely to excessive moulding, relief from the dangerous outside pressure certainly would be desirable but, unfortunately, application of the forceps and extraction will actually augment this pressure and the operation result in more harm than good.

Summarizing briefly all the new information gained in the past three years concerning intracranial birth injuries we can state:

A fact, previously only suspected, now is definitely established, namely, that cerebral injuries of various character and different degree occur by far more often than was suggested by the discovery of lacerations of dural septa in approximately one half of the infants either stillborn or dying within the first few days of life.

We understand more clearly than heretofore the relation of such lesions to anomalies of physical and mental development of the child.

We should consider with greater concern every artificial method of hastening the expulsion of the fetus, especially if we know it to be premature. We should remember the unquestionable fact that haste of any kind must imply a risk to the child far greater than the possible benefit of a quicker delivery.

**Injuries of Vertebral Column and Spinal Cord.**—Primary breech labors, and foot extractions subsequent to version prove not much less dangerous to the integrity of the vertebral column and spinal cord than we have shown these methods of delivery to be to the brain and especially to the septa of the dura mater. However, these vertebral injuries are discovered only if the autopsy includes a careful dissection of the column, which is yet to become the routine practice.

The high frequency of damage to the spinal column is clearly evidenced in the report of Pierson from the Sloane Hospital for Women. Analyzing the deliveries of the past three years only, he found in 142 viable primary breech labors an infant mortality of 12 per cent; in 87 viable version and breech deliveries of 26 per cent. Of 36 cases carefully investigated at necropsy a spinal cord hemorrhage was noted in 47 per cent, fractured vertebræ found in 38 per cent. There was an intracranial hemorrhage present in 44 per cent, though it was extensive only in 25 per cent. He calculates that the probable cause of death in these 36 cases was: Trauma alone in 56 per cent; asphyxia alone probably in only 5 per cent; while both trauma and asphyxia might have accounted for death in the remaining 39 per cent.

Crothers also emphasizes the true but regrettable fact that injuries of the spinal cord are only rarely diagnosed by the obstetrician though decidedly often discovered by the pathologist. Disability from such accidents is but seldom recognized by those who see older children.

Serious damage to the spinal cord then would not seem consistent with continued life. After an extensive experimental study of the problem Crothers, however, arrived at the conclusion that in breech labors another factor, outside the cord injury itself, must be the element which is really responsible for the infant's death, and suggests herniation of the cerebellum and medulla through the foramen magnum, as mentioned in preceding pages. Under normal conditions in breech labors the medulla is guarded from harmful pressure by the tentorium which modifies and controls the force imposed upon the vertex from above. Rupture of the tentorium and a combination of pressure and pull are likely to lead to this dangerous herniation of the medulla because of increased intracranial pressure concurrent with actual decrease of intraspinal pressure.

Belfrage and Kohlbry among others describe the later consequences of such spinal birth injuries, the latter detailing a case which exhibits the almost typical sequence of subsequent pathologic manifestations leading to death: At birth a paralysis of the sphincter of the bladder; at the age of 3½ months, a marked pyuria; death at 9 months. Postmortem findings: Hydronephrosis, pyelonephritis, complete degeneration of all tracts in the cervical portion of the cord.

**Brachial Birth Palsy.**—A thorough discussion of all the various aspects of obstetrical brachial paralysis will be found in a paper of Boorstein. From a study of 64 patients he concludes that the condition is due to stretching or tearing of the cervical roots of the brachial plexus. Almost always the condition is found associated with a history of difficult labor or artificial delivery. The right arm is affected more often than the left, and bilateral affections are very infrequent. The upper arm type, caused by injury of the suprascapular and fifth and sixth cervical nerves, is more common than the lower arm type. If these cases are treated early and properly one can expect good recovery of all mild cases in 3 or 4 months, but severe cases will require 6 to 7 months. When no result is obtained by conservative measures within 4 months, nerve operations are indicated which later have to be followed with orthopedic treatment.

Froelich also feels that the prognosis in general is good and that the palsy only exceptionally leads to a permanent flail joint of the shoulder. Proper treatment, in his opinion, consists in immediate immobilization of the affected arm in a position in which all traction strain is taken from the roots of the plexus, and which at the same time is antagonistic to the contraction of the unaffected muscles.

Brachial paralysis in the majority of instances, according to Schubert, is due to a primary plexus injury although at times anomalies of the central nervous system contribute to its etiology. The fairly common observation of brachial palsy combined with other congenital deformities due to developmental defects, speaks in favor of such an assumption.

Another case of that rather rare type of isolated paralysis of the radial nerve in the newborn is placed on record by Treu. The condition was noticed two days after an easy forceps extraction. An x-ray examination failed to reveal any bone injury. On the outer surface of the upper arm there could be seen a pressure mark on the skin, the size of a penny, which was infiltrated and situated approximately just above the musculospiral nerve, where it emerges between the brachioradialis and the brachialis anticus muscles. This part of the upper arm seemingly had been pressed against the promontory owing to a deflexed attitude of the head.

**Torticollis.**—Schubert suggests that the congenital wry-neck is caused by peripheral trophoneurotic disturbances due to cerebral defects. Weil objects to this view and advances evidence for his own contention that the shortening of the sternomastoid muscle is the outcome of abnormal pressure brought on by an anomalous intrauterine posture. This explanation of the etiology of torticollis is most convincingly established in a case carefully studied and described by Stern.

**Injuries of the Eye.**—The ophthalmoscopic study by Jacobs of the eye-grounds of 157 infants within 24 hours after birth fully confirms previous statements concerning the frequency of retinal hemorrhages. They were found by him in 12.1 per cent of all the newborn babies he examined. Extravasation of blood appeared either in the form of radial streaks about the disk or surrounding the latter in circular form. He emphasizes that such traumatic retinal lesions frequently result in permanent changes.

Doerfler noticed in an infant an exophthalmus within 24 hours after labor. On the seventh day the eye was bulging far out so that the lids could not close over it. A suspected orbital fracture was excluded by x-ray examination. Two days later there were observed clonic contractions of left arm and left leg, followed next day by contractions also of the right leg. Although a lumbar puncture yielded a perfectly clear fluid and the baby finally recovered, Doerfler feels certain that the exophthalmus in this instance was caused by an intracranial hemorrhage.

Of unusual interest is the practically unique observation recorded by Gerdes. Immediately after an easy low forceps extraction the left bulb was seen to lie outside the palpebral fissure. Slight pressure replaced it into the socket. In looking for the possible cause of this apparently serious injury, it was found that comparatively slight pressure against the frontal bone just above the supraorbital arch immediately caused the luxation to recur. Again the eyeball was replaced with the greatest ease. The remarkable feature of this case is that Gerdes, 18 years after this accident, had the opportunity to meet this infant as a fullgrown, healthy girl. She had not the slightest visual disturbance. Frontal bone and orbital ridge were normal. In confessing to the parents that he had hidden from them the occurrence of this accident, which at the time almost had induced him to cut the eye off since it seemed to hang only on a few tissue shreds, he was told that this same accident had also occurred later when again the eyeball had been easily pushed back into the socket. In this case the luxation of the bulbus oculi unquestionably was the result of only normal pressure of a forceps blade against an unusually elastic frontal bone.

**Injuries of the Ear.**—Reference already has been made to hemorrhages in the vestibulary apparatus described by Voss, Berberich, Wiechers, etc. Hartog believes that so-called congenital deaf-mutism more often than is usually suspected is due to actual injury of the hearing mechanism in labor. In other cases the damage may consist merely in hemorrhage into the labyrinth or cochlea, caused by undue pressure over the temporal bone, especially from awkward application of the forceps.

**Injuries of the Scalp.**—Fueth demonstrates in detail how a ring-like pressure necrosis of the soft tissues on the child's head can result from the spasmodic contraction of the cervix about it. Indeed, in his own case and in another quoted from literature this same condition appeared in two successive labors, with no pelvic contraction nor any other possible cause for the injury. Analyzing several other cases of this sort, as reported in literature, he notes that in all of them labors were prolonged and the membranes had ruptured prematurely. In several of these instances it could be shown that it was a spasm of the internal rather than of the external os which occasioned the injury and in his opinion this explanation holds true for all cases. Several of the infants died as the result of an infection of the necrotic area.

Such traumatic lesions must be clearly differentiated from congenital skin defects at least for the one reason, pointed out by Moeller, that the patients seem prone to interpret the congenital lesions as injuries produced by the attending physician or midwife. In some instances, he emphasizes, a clear distinction between these two types might be impossible. Newmann, dwelling on this same point, stresses the necessity of differentiating either type from luetic ulcers. In his opinion, at least in the two cases described by him, the defects were congenital, the result of amniotic adhesions. Walz doubts that this commonly assumed etiology holds true for the majority of congenital defects. He believes that they, like harelip or syndactylism, etc., more likely have an endogenous origin, and exhibit the following etiologic progressive stages: Acrania, hemicrania, encephalocele and, least marked, merely a skin defect. That they occasionally are found associated with anomalies of the bony skull roof is pointed out by Neumann in another paper.

Such bone defects, like the skin defects, not only are unjustly interpreted as traumatic injuries and blamed on the attending physician, but might prove mystifying during labor in diagnosing accurately the presentation.

Heidler discusses this entire problem in detail. In his own case, the full term, though somewhat small, child had a sharply defined skin defect over one parietal bone. Underneath this skin defect also the bone was missing, and more anteriorly the parietal bone was soft and of a spongy consistence. When the infant was four weeks old a severe hemorrhage occurred from this area which finally was controlled by tight compression with bandages. Later, bleeding reappeared whenever the child was crying. At the age of two months a meningitis was soon followed by death. A partial autopsy showed that the bleeding originated from the longitudinal sinus. The author compares the various striking similarities between this case and one recorded previously by Moeller, and discussing the etiology of such defects he expresses the belief that it is unlikely they are caused by amniotic adhesions but more probably represent primary inhibitions of development of a still unknown etiology.

**Fractures and Luxations.**—A few newer observations of intrauterine fractures of long bones of the fetus, seemingly caused by an external trauma, are worthy of citation.

In the case of Genova a fracture in the lower third of the left leg was at the time of birth in the state of advanced healing with a marked angle at the site of the break. In his opinion the fracture was produced by an accident sustained in the seventh month of pregnancy, but its occurrence favored by a coincident oligohydramnion, since the latter condition exposes the fetus more directly to traumatization by an external force.

Most remarkable is a case reported by Rouvier to the Obstetric Society of Paris. Though evidently full term, the infant weighed only 1710 Gms. It showed multiple fractures of the extremities resulting in angular bending, especially of both limbs. He accepts as a perfectly plausible explanation of this striking deformity the fact that the patient, with the definite intention to produce an abortion, had worn from the seventh month of pregnancy a band around the abdomen, tight enough to cause partial necrosis of the skin underneath it. The continued constriction, in his belief, accounts for the small size of the infant and must have caused the fractures because the band came to lie just over the lower extremities with the fetus in a vertex presentation.

Decidedly less convincing as an example of fetal traumatization by external force proves a case described by Fink. A woman, about seven to eight months pregnant, fell from a bicycle. She gave birth, 48 hours later, to a premature child, born in a breech presentation, which soon died. Fink insists that the fetal subdural hematoma, discovered at autopsy, must have been caused by the accident in spite of the fact that the skull bones were found intact.

The entire question of fractures occurring during birth is thoroughly discussed in a thesis by Stinz.

While, in general, injuries of the upper extremities during the management of the aftercoming head are fairly common, among them only rarely is found a luxation of the elbow, *e.g.*, in the case of Kahn. The existence of the injury in this premature infant was discovered only on the fifth day on account of a swelling. Reposition became impossible because the median epicondylus of the humerus had been detached.

The origin of luxation of the knee-joint, Sachs points out, has never been satisfactorily determined. The theory of abnormal intrauterine direct pressure on account of scantiness of amniotic fluid certainly could not apply to his own case. Sometimes the condition is due to an abnormal relaxation of the joint capsule and this factor might account for the occasional observation of such a luxation in several children of the same mother, or in several joints of the same child. Potel thought of a primary retraction of the quadriceps. Drehman assumed that during intrauterine growth the affected leg had been maintained in an abnormal posture by the foot being caught under the chin or in the axilla of the fetus. Sachs concludes his paper with the assurance of fairly good prognosis if treatment is started early.

**Hemorrhages in the Suprarenal Glands.**—It affords great satisfaction to realize that newer knowledge concerning birth injuries tends to reduce visibly the number of instances in which even autopsy fails to reveal the cause of death in stillborn or very young infants. An improved technic in the examination of the head, a careful dissection of the spinal column, especially of its cervical portion, a study of the spinal cord or of the pons, etc., as shown in preceding pages, furnishes a great deal of unexpected information. The proper routine autopsy on a newborn infant should include as well the inspection and study of the adrenals.

They are not infrequently injured in labor and particularly by manipulations in which the baby is grasped around the waistline.

Vallois and Roume saw a full-term baby, without any difficulty borne by a quartipara, collapse on the second day and die on the third day postpartum. The only pathologic finding discovered at necropsy to explain the death consisted in hemorrhages in the adrenals. In a case of Cornil and Tonzard a spontaneously born child, asphyxiated but successfully resuscitated, died eight hours later. Both adrenals were found completely torn apart by large hematomas so that only a narrow edge of suprarenal tissue was remaining. There were no other noteworthy autopsy findings. The fatal injury must have been produced during the manipulations in resuscitation.

The report of Browne, comprising a series of 400 cases of stillbirths and neonatal deaths, contains 27 instances of suprarenal hemorrhages, only six of these children being born alive but dying soon, the latest four days postpartum. Usually the capsule of one or both glands is found distended by the hematomas in the medulla, and only occasionally the extravasated blood had burst into the free abdominal cavity. Browne points to the noteworthy fact that this accident seemingly is about 22 times as likely to happen with breech as with vertex deliveries, three times as likely in premature as in full term infants.

To Corcoran and Strauss seemingly belongs credit for the first successful operation on a suprarenal hemorrhage of a newborn infant. This baby, weighing 5575 Gms., was borne by a quartipara. It became sick on the fourth day. An abdominal mass over to the left side was discovered the next day and the baby operated upon the same afternoon. A hematoma, the size of a fetal head, was removed from the intact adrenal capsule and but one bleeding point ligated. The infant recovered and remained well—a remarkable proof of good surgical judgment, an encouraging example of the efficacy of prompt and proper interference for a most serious type of birth injury.

## LITERATURE

Ballance and Ballance. Lancet, London, 1922, 203:1109.
Bartram. Ztschr. f. Geburtsh. u. Gynäk. Stuttg., 1922, 84:34.
Behrendt. Fortschr. d. Med., Berlin, 1922, 40:454.
Beitzke. Deutsche med. Wchnschr., Leipz., 1922, 48:1040.
Belfrage. Acta Paediatrica, Upsala, 1923, 3:91.
Berberich and Wieders. Ztschr. f. Kinderh., 1924, 38:59.
Boorstein. J. Am. M. Ass., Chicago, 1924, 82:862.
Idem. J. Bone & Joint Surg., 1923, 21:778.

Brady. Medical Clinics of North America, 1923-1924, 7:1453.
Browne. Brit. M. J., London, Sept. 30, 1922, 590.
Burhans and Gerstenberger. J. Am. M. Ass., Chicago, 1923, 80:604.
Cameron and Osman. Brit. M. J., March 3, 1923, 363.
Cameron. Lancet, London, 1923, 205:1292.
Capon. J. Obst. & Gynæc. Brit. Emp., 1922, 29:572.
Conkey. Arch. Pediat., New York, 1923, 40:239.
Corcoran and Strauss. J. Am. M. Ass., Chicago, 1924, 82:626.
Cornil and Tonzard. Bull. et mém. Soc. anat. de Par., 1923, 93:370.
Crothers. Am. J. M. Sc., Phila., 1923, 165:94.
Idem. Surg., Gynec. & Obst., Chicago, 1923, 37:790.
Cruickshank. Lancet, London, 1923, 204:836.
De Angelis. Pediatria, Naples, 1922, 30:1107.
Doerfler. München. med. Wchnschr., 1922, 69:1117.
Dollinger. Deutsche med. Wchnschr., Leipz., 1922, 48:1726.
Ehrenfest. Illinois M. J., 1923, 44:20.
Idem. Am. J. Dis. Child., Chicago, 1923, 26:503.
Falls. J. Am. M. Ass., Chicago, 1923, 80:678.
Fink. Monatschr. f. Geburtsh. u. Gynaek., Berl., 1922, 59:264.
Fischer. Schweiz. med. Wchnschr., 1924, 54:905.
Frey. Zentralbl. f. Gynäk., Leipz., 1924, 48:947.
Froelich. Rev. de chir., Par., 1921, 59:419.
Fueth. Ztschr. f. Geburtsh. u. Gynäk., Stuttg., 1923, 86:633.
Gamper. Monatschr. f. Geburtsh. u. Gynaek., Berl., 1923, 64:296.
Genova. Ann. di ostet., 1923, 45:294.
Gerdes. München med. Wchnschr., 1924, 71:274.
Gordon. Am. J. Obst. & Gynec., St. Louis, 1924, 7:462.
Idem. Am. J. Dis. Child., Chicago, 1924, 27:303.
Greenwood. J. Obst. & Gynæc. Brit. Emp., 1924, 31:611.
Hamill. Medical Clinics of North America, 1923-1924, 7:407.
Hartog. Nederlandsch Tijdschr. voor Verloskunde en Gynaek., 1924, 29:256.
Heidler. Wien. klin. Wchnschr., 1924, 38:114.
Henkel. Zentralbl. f. Gynäk., Leipz., 1922, 46:129.
Holland. J. Obst. & Gynæc. Brit. Emp., 1922, 29:531.
Idem. Brit. M. J., Sept. 30, 1922, 588.
Jacobs. J. Am. M. Ass., Chicago, 1924, 83:1641.
Kahn. Zentralbl. f. Gynäk., Leipz., 1922, 46:1318.
Kaiser. N. York M. J., 1922, 116:156.
Keene. Lancet, Lond., 1923, 204:1054.
Kirby. Arch. of Ophth., N. Y., 1923, 52:452.

Kirkwood and Meyers. Lancet, Lond., 1923, 205:65.
Kohlbry. Am. J. Dis. Child., Chicago, 1923, 26:242.
Levinson. Abt's Pediatrics, Saunders, Phila., Vol. II, 120.
Moeller. Acta Gynaecologica Scandinavica, Helsingfors, 1924, 2:144.
Munro and Eustis. Am. J. Dis. Child., Chicago, 1922, 24:272.
Neumann. Zentralbl. f. Gynäk., Leipz., 1924, 48:571, 628.
Patrick and Levy. J. Am. M. Ass., Chicago, 1924, 82:375.
Pierson. Surg., Gynec. & Obst., Chicago, 1923, 37:802.
Raisz. Abstract, Zentralbl. f. Gynäk., Leipz., 1922, 46:524.
Reis. Surg., Gynec. & Obst., Chicago, 1923, 37:206.
Rouvier. Bull. Soc. d'obst. et de gynéc. de Par., 1924, 13:241.
Sachs. Ztschr. f. Geburtsh. u. Gynäk., Stuttg., 1924, 87:639.
Saenger. Monatschr. f. Geburtsh. u. Gynaek., Berl., 1924, 65:258.
Santner. Monatschr. f. Geburtsh. u. Gynaek., Berl., 1923, 62:289.
Schele. Monatschr. f. Kinderh., 1923, 26:43.
Schubert. Deutsche Ztschr. f. Chir., 1922, 170:343.
Schwartz. Ztschr. f. d. ges. Neurol, u. Psychiat, 1924, 90:263.
Idem. Deutsche med. Wchnschr., Berl., 1924, 50:1375.
Sharpe. J. Am. M. Ass., Chicago, 1923, 81:620.
Sharpe and Maclaire. Surg., Gynec. & Obst., Chicago, 1924, 38:200.
Idem. Am. J. Obst. & Gynec., St. Louis, 1924, 8:172.
Siegmund. München. med. Wchnschr., 1923, 70:137.
Stern. Monatschr. f. Geburtsh. u. Gynaek., Berl., 1924, 65:179.
Stern and Schwartz. Klin. Wchnschr., Berl., 1924, 3:931.
Still. Lancet, Lond., 1923, 204:431.
Stinz. Inaugural Dissertation, Liepzig, 1923.
Stroehm. Zentralbl. f. Gynäk., Leipz., 1923, 67:922.
Treu. Zentralbl. f. Gynäk., Leipz., 1924, 68:1018.
Vallois and Roume. Bull. Soc. d'obst. et de gynéc. de Par., 1923, 21:1.
Vogel. Ztschr. f. Geburtsh. u. Gynäk., Stuttg., 1924, 88:158.
Voss. Ztschr. f. Hals-Nasen u. Ohrenkrankheiten, 1923, 6, Congress-bericht.
Walz. Monatschr. f. Geburtsh. u. Gynaek., Berl., 1924, 65:167.
Weil. Klin. Wchnschr., Berl., 1922, 1:1260.
Ylppoe. Klin. Wchnschr., Berl., 1922, 1:1241.
Idem. Ztschr. f. Kinderh., 1924, 38:32.

# PELVIC NEOPLASMS

FRANK W. LYNCH, M.D., AND A. F. MAXWELL, M.D.

## APPENDIX

In the three years which have elapsed since the publication of the manuscript on *Pelvic Neoplasms,* there has accumulated a very considerable literature. While most of it is centered about carcinoma of the uterus, and the relative values of Roentgen ray, radium, and surgery, as therapeutic agents, there have been many contributions on other subjects of such value as to warrant this cursory review of the literature.

## BENIGN TUMORS OF THE OUTLET

**Fibroma of the Vulva.**—Most of the literature on this subject is confined to case reports and no one has attempted a review comparable to the splendid contribution which Leonard made in 1917. Ferguson,[1] in 1924, described a tumor which had developed in two years from the left labium into a pendulous growth two feet two inches long, and with a diameter of three inches at the lower pole. It proved to be a telangiectatic fibroma. It falls in the first group of Leonard's classification and appears to have arisen shortly after a fall two years before. The patient had had an operation for uterine fibroids five years previously. The large myxoma of the labium majus, reported by Fisher, in 1919, is pictured in Taussig's monograph Diseases of the Vulva in this series. Fullerton,[2] in February, 1925, describes a fibroid in the vestibule. Tumors in this location are rarely seen. In Leonard's comprehensive review of 131 cases, there were only five tumors in this location. Attwenger,[3] in 1923, describes a fibroma of the clitoris which grew completely in only seven weeks. The tumor was pear-shaped; dissection proved that it rose from the caput clitoris.

Taussig,[4] who has made so many valuable contributions to the pathology of the vulva, in 1923 described an angioma which developed from a congenital nevus. Most of the hemangiomas have been found in children, yet even they are very rare.

**Lipoma of the Vulva.**—Lovelace,[5] in 1923, reported a lipoma which originated from the left labium. It hung down to the patient's knees like an apron, weighed 44 pounds and was said to have developed in 3½ years. The patient was five feet six inches tall, and weighed 200 pounds. The photograph, which will be found on page 125 of Taussig's monograph of this series, does not show the origin as given by the author, but looks like a lipoma which has arisen from the fat of the lower abdominal wall. Lipomas of the abdominal wall often stretch out and have a rather broad thin pedicle, although they usually arise in the abdomen higher than shown in the illustration. Lovelace, however, is conversant with the large lipomas of the lower abdominal wall, since he alludes to the case of Christopherson in 1906, in which an Arab of about 65 years had such a fatty tumor in the lower abdomen, the skin hanging down from the umbilicus to the middle of the thigh like a bag, enclosing a mass of fat and becoming continuous behind with the abdominal skin again over the pubis. If the tumor of Lovelace is really vulvar and not as it appears in the photograph, it is very much larger than any other case on record, since there is reason to believe that the Balls-Headley tumor quoted in our text as 24 pounds weighed in reality only two pounds. This tumor is quoted in the literature usually as 21 pounds. The tumor of Steigele has been quoted as 101 pounds. We accepted it as ten pounds. The errors in the literature occurred because of the peculiar character of type used in printing the Balls-Headley article in the Australian Medical Journal in 1888, in which the characters for the letter "l" and the figure "1" are identical, and because there was no spacing between the numerals and the symbols "lbs." Lovelace reviews the literature of fatty tumors of the vulva and finds 45 cases.

**Sweat Glands of the Vulva.**—Schellekens,[6] in 1923, describes a case of this rare tumor, which proved to be an adenoma, situated in the left labia of a woman of 39.

## MALIGNANT TUMORS OF THE OUTLET

**Carcinoma of the Vulva.**—Taussig[7] has covered so completely this subject in his monograph in this series that there is little to add at the present time. The newer literature consists of case reports, many of which are only citations in discussions in gynecologic societies. For the most part, they record experiences with radium or the Roentgen ray while others urge the very close relationship between leukoplakia and the cancer and insist upon treatment of leukoplakia on the basis of its being a precancerous condition.

Our review of the subject promotes a profound pessimism as to the present day curability of the usual run of vulval carcinoma since the disease occurs usually in the old and feeble, who seek treatment only when the growth is far advanced.

There is no doubt but that radical surgery will cure selected cases. This is well proved by Taussig's report in 1923. Three of his nine cases treated by *radical* surgery remained well for more than five years. One was lost track of after two years when she was free of recurrence. Taussig's review proves his belief that *radical surgery will cure more than 30 per cent of the cases operated,* provided a radical lymph gland dissection is done coincident with the wide removal of the primary growth. Yet surgery as usually performed is not radical and rarely, if ever, cures, and it is an open question whether it is worth while, if the general profession continues to treat these growths. The pessimistic view of the condition given in our texts is based upon reports from university clinics, where presumably surgery was more radical than in general hands.

Our individual observations convince us that cancer of the vulva, although comparatively rare, occurs far more frequently than is evidenced by the literature. Moreover, it is treated usually by general practitioners whose therapy consists of simple excision, which rarely offers any chance of

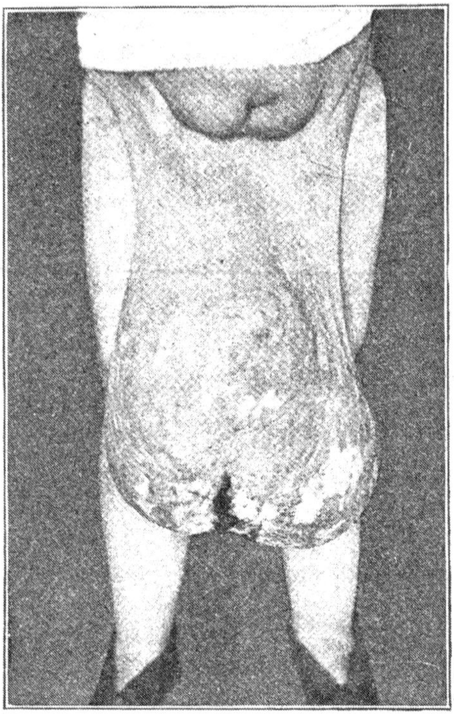

FIG. 1.—HUGE LIPOMA OF VULVA. (Lovelace, *J. Am. M. Ass.*)

cure. Since the prognosis of carcinoma of the vulva is sufficiently gloomy, even after a *radical* dissection, and the simple excision is not even palliative, we believe a sentiment should be created to discredit strongly any but truly radical surgical procedures and to advocate those only after the tumor region and the groin have been rayed either by radium or the modern Roentgen ray.

Furthermore, we believe that the majority of cases will be treated equally successfully by the modern Roentgen ray and by radium, either alone or in combination. Since the appearance of the text, the modern Roentgen ray has come to occupy a definite field in the therapy of malignant tumors, and far surpasses even the most favorable results obtained by the older machines. The value of radium treatment is well established and there are several reports of five-year cures. A number of observers have used radium emanations in fine glass needles known as "bare tubes," each tube containing 0.5 mc. or 1 mc. buried at least 1 cm. in depth and ½-1 cm. apart. The method is illustrated in Taussig's monograph. We have had good local results in this manner but without cures, because the cases had marked inguinal involvement. Several writers record their experiences with radium but have not followed their cases sufficiently long to talk of cure. Bailey and Bagg,[8] in 1921, recorded ten cancers of the vulva treated by a combination of radium and surgery. The tumors were first treated with massive doses of radium, after which the lymphatics of the groin were dissected out and the wound was needled with a number of bare tubes each containing .5 mc. radium element placed ½ cm. apart. Keene,[9] in a discussion of Bailey and Bagg's paper, alludes to 19 malignant tumors of the vulva or vagina which were treated by radium in the gynecological service of the University of Pennsylvania. Seventeen were carcinomas and two were chorionepitheliomas. The cases as vulval or vaginal growths were not separated. All were radiated. The two chorionepithelioma were alive and well five and six years after treatment. Four of the 17 other cases were known to have survived, one for one and a half years, one for two and a half years, one for three years, and one between five and six years. E. Zweifel,[10] in 1922, reported 29 cases of vulvar carcinoma treated in the University Clinic in Munich by radium. One case was symptom-free seven years after the treatment. Schmitz,[11] in 1924, cites a vulvar carcinoma cured for five years by radium.

While the procedure of Bailey and Bagg cannot be duplicated by many men, since it involves an enormous amount of radium, there are enough modern Roentgen ray machines scattered through nearly every town to warrant treatment by the gamma ray. Radium, moreover, is nearly universally employed in the United States and even 100 Mgms. of the radium element will suffice for treatment.

**Carcinoma of the Female Urethra.**—Carcinoma of the female urethra may be primary or secondary. It is a rare disease, although there is no doubt that it occurs much more often than is indicated in the literature. Many men, however, of extensive experience may have seen only two or three cases. Ehrendorfer, in 1899, quoted 27 cases. Yet O'Neil,[12] in 1921, was able to collect but 68 cases and Venot and Parcelier, later in the same year, reviewed only 87 cases. Keene, in 1921, mentioned 6 cases seen in the Gynecologic Clinic of the University of Pennsylvania. Since then Pomeroy, O'Conor, and several others have described individual cases. We have seen only one case in a series of nearly 400 pelvic cancers.

The primary tumor may arise from the mucous membrane of the urethra or from Littre's or Skene's glands. It often arises from a chronic inflammatory area; more rarely from a caruncle. There are two major types; the polypoid or everting, and the ulcerative or infiltrating form. Beginning usually in the canal near the external orifice, the tumor tends to grow outward since the structure of the urethra resists invasion for a considerable time. The growth, therefore, soon appears at the external meatus where it spreads to the surrounding tissues. The appearance of the tumor varies considerably accordingly as the carcinoma is or is not superimposed upon a preëxisting infection. The tumors arising from infected areas are usually of a slower type of growth than those which are frankly carcinomatous from the start. The tumor may be of squamous cell or of cylindrical cell epithelium. It metastasizes through the lymphatics along both the anterior and posterior surface of the pubis to the glands in the groin or the pelvis. Many have called attention to the late involvement of glands. Venot and Parcelier [13] found that they were not enlarged or appeared grossly normal in two-thirds of cases.

The secondary carcinoma of the urethra is usually a metastasis from a cancer of the uterus.

The disease may be mistaken for an ulcerative infiltrating erosion of syphilis from which it can be differentiated by the presence of spirochetes or by biopsy. The Wassermann reaction may give a clue. The superficial vestibular urethral form of carcinoma may also be confused with tuberculosis, although the latter usually presents a more even surface without the same tendency to infiltration. An ulcerating fibroid of the urethra may also be confused with carcinoma, although the former is more isolated and can be readily shelled out of its capsule. Older writers urge biopsy since there has been much difficulty in distinguishing the transition of the simple adenoma into the malignant adenocarcinoma. The suggestion is rational only if it can be done by diathermy or the cautery knife.

Radium appears the most likely method of treatment at the present time although there are very few cases reported in the literature. Shaw,[16] in 1923, reported two cases well three years after radium. Schmitz,[11] in December, 1924, reported two out of five five-year cures. Radium did not help our case, a woman of 54, with rather advanced growth, who died within the year. Surgical procedures have removed the urethra even to within 1 cm. of the neck of the bladder and dissected out the lymphatics on both sides of the symphysis. It does not seem a reasonable method if the growth is advanced, since the patient is likely to lose urinary control, when the operation merely adds to her suffering. Only two of Ehrendorfer's 27 cases were free from recurrence as long as three years. The majority of cases succumbed within a year, although R. Peterson had one which survived for five years and Vineberg one three years without relapse. O'Conor,[15] in 1924, reported a case treated by diathermy and radium. The local cure was perfect although the ultimate prognosis was hopeless because of extensive glandular involvement. The urinary control remained good even in advanced cases of the disease. The literature abounds with cases retaining urinary control even after extensive surgical procedures. When radium is inserted in the urethra, the greatest care must be taken to hold it in place. The same holds for plaques which are applied locally to the growth. We have seen a case where a burn followed displacement of the radium capsules.

**Carcinoma of Bartholin Gland.**—This tumor is undoubtedly rare, yet the literature does not properly express the frequency, since vulvar growths are usually seen by men in general practice who do not report them and who may be content merely with their removal. Falls,[17] in 1923, reviews the cases of this rare tumor, collecting 17, only three of which were in America. The cases were nearly equally divided between squamous cell epithelioma and adenocarcinoma. Falls' case was treated by radical surgery, radium, and Roentgen ray and remained without recurrence for 14 months thereafter, when the case was reported. Casler, in the discussion of Falls' case, alludes to an unreported adenocarcinoma seen in Kelly's clinic in the Johns Hopkins Hospital. The patient entered because of a prolapse of the uterus, at which time a small tumor about the size of the end of a thumb was found in the labia. Treatment consisted merely in excision, since it was not believed to be malignant until the routine laboratory examination. The patient remains alive and perfectly well 16 years later, probably because the growth was so early that it had created neither symptoms nor metastasis, a condition that is seldom duplicated.

Casler also alludes to a papillary cystadenoma which showed malignant changes in several places. The case was also seen in the Johns Hopkins Clinic. Falls' cases were limited to primary growths. Pfeiffer,[18] in 1923, described a secondary cancer in the Bartholin gland, a metastasis from a cancer primary in the uterus. Pfeiffer records this as the second case of the kind on record.

**Sarcoma of the Vulva.**—R. Veit,[19] in 1924, reported a non-pigmented sarcoma of the vulva which originated, he believed, either in the supporting tissue of the Bartholin gland, or from the connective tissue stroma. He found in the literature only two other cases of similar origin, one recorded by Hofmeier in 1920 and the other by A. Bluhm in 1904. His review suggests that there are only about 50 cases recorded of non-pigmented sarcoma. The only one which began during pregnancy was described by Neuwirth in 1917. It began in the third month but the patient did not die until two years later. Veit's case was treated with surgery combined with the modern Roentgen ray. The result is not known since the case was followed only for eight months, at which time there was no recurrence. Casler, in the discussion of Falls' paper on carcinoma of the Bartholin gland, alludes to a sarcoma of the Bartholin gland seen in Kelly's clinic in the Johns Hopkins Hospital.

## MALIGNANT TUMORS OF THE VAGINA

**Carcinoma of the Vagina.**—There are a number of individual case reports in the literature of this rare tumor, although no systematic review is attempted. Bailey and Bagg, in 1921, reported 18 cases, all of which were treated by radium. The tumors were all primary with two exceptions. There is no discussion as to cure since the longest period of observation was but two years. Stacy,[20] in 1922, records 21 cases treated by radium. The cases were not followed long enough to permit of discussion as to cure. It is of interest, however, to find that 14 of the 21 cases had some follow-up record. Seven lived for periods varying from five months to nearly four years; of the seven which died, one lived two years and four months and two others for more than a year.

Keene, in 1921, urges the greatest care in radiating carcinoma of the rectovaginal septum since fistulas very frequently result. This distressing complication occurred in three of the 17 carcinomas of the vagina or vulva treated in Clark's clinic in the University of Pennsylvania. Fistulas of the rectovaginal septum occur more frequently than in the bladder wall. While fistulas often follow radiation, it is well to recall that they are often seen as a direct result of extension of the disease. Even with the possibility of fistula formation, treatment with radium is a logical procedure. Surgery certainly creates greater complications and deformities. Because of the chance of distressing sequelæ, it seems logical at present to urge that cases with this dread disease be sent to men well versed in the radium treatment so that they may treat the growth locally with radium and spray the pelvis with the modern Roentgen ray for metastasis. It seems logical also to urge the needling of the local tumor with tubes of radium emanation, each of 1 mc. placed 1 cm. apart.

**Sarcoma of the Vagina.**—Dellepiane,[21] in 1924, reported a spindle-celled sarcoma of the vagina found in a nulliparous woman of 21 years of age. She had been married two years. Symptoms had occurred for six months and consisted in painful micturition and bloody vaginal discharge. A nodular, somewhat necrotic mass extended well into the posterior vaginal wall and infiltrated adjacent tissues. The cervix was not involved. The case was treated with the modern Roentgen ray with local and subjective improvement for the seven months during which the case was under observation.

## BENIGN TUMORS OF THE UTERUS

**Lipoma of Uterus.**—Schleussner [22] reports a case which he cites as the seventeenth lipomatous tumor on record. Four occurred as cervical polyps, his and 12 others were tumors of the body of the uterus. His and six others are simple lipoma. The other ten are lipomyoma.

**Adenomyoma.**—*Frequency.*—There were 211 adenomyoma in 3388 fibroids reported from the Mayo Clinic, 6.43 per cent. There were five cases in the fallopian tubes.

*Etiology.*—The theory of Cullen that adenomyoma were extensions of uterine mucosa into fibroid tissue for a long time served to explain this great group of tumors. The mucosa functioned as uterine mucosa, gave decidual reactions in pregnancy, and secreted blood during menstruation. The extensions of the endometrium were also proved by serial sections in 55 of 56 tumors. The theory appeared to lack only a reason for the mucosal infiltration. This defect was presently supplied by von Franqué, Legueu, Marie, and others who saw it as a result of chronic inflammation.

Others believed that it was closely dependent upon the changes incidental to gestation. The limitations of the theory became evident only with the recognition of the "ectopic" adenomyoma. While it accounted satisfactorily for the uterine tumors, it failed to account for the ectopic adenomyoma of the pelvis, such as adenomyoma of the ovary, or those in the pockets of the pelvis as on the uterosacral ligaments, or the tumors of the rectovaginal septum.

The theory of von Recklinghausen also had some supporters. It advanced the view that adenomyoma of the uterus sprang from fetal rests of wolffian origin, a belief built purely on theory and not susceptible of proof. It accounted satisfactorily for the adenomyoma in the uterine horns but failed to explain tumors in other locations. Many argued against it on the ground that it was illogical. Some claimed, as R. Meyer, that the tubules have no resemblance to the wolffian duct or any of its derivatives, while others argued that the embryonic areas never came close enough together to account for the tumor in adult life.

Admitting the possibility of the theory, it was soon found that other explanations could account equally well even for the tumors near the horns. Von Franqué demonstrated that epithelial infiltration was a frequent finding in chronic salpingitis of tuberculous type. Lubarsch, in 1902, and R. Meyer, in 1903, found that this phenomenon is not limited to tuberculous salpingitis but could occur with any tubal inflammation.

This inflammatory theory soon took on wider proportions. The cause of the epithelial proliferation was taken as a preëxistent inflammation. Granulation tissue, areas of round-cell infiltration, and proliferating connective tissues were all held to be permeable to a benign epithelial infiltration. The proliferation of the epithelium was interpreted as a reaction to aid in the repair of damage done by the inflammation. Meyer used the term epithelial heterotopy to characterize the non-malignant invasion of the epithelial membrane. He felt that any epithelial structure could take on this function in the presence of inflammation. Orth had described a similar process about the suppurative follicles in amebic dysentery. Ziegler had described the same condition in abscess of the bowel. Richter had found like processes in ileocecal ulcers in tuberculosis. The theory now advocated chiefly by Meyer explained satisfactorily, as did Cullen's, the intrauterine adenomyoma.

Meyer explained ectopic adenomyoma by the theory that Iwanoff advocated in 1898 to account for adenomyoma. Ivanoff believed that the glandular structures were derived from the peritoneal serosa by the process of metaplasia. Under the stimulus of inflammation, the peritoneal epithelium proliferates and sends down bands of cell-buds into the subjacent tissue. These proliferate and form branching tubular processes, the cells of which become indistinguishable from columnar epithelium derived from true mucous membrane. The connective tissue changes its character and becomes the cytogenous tissue so characteristic of the adenoma.

Meyer believes all adenomyoma arise on an inflammatory base and the epithelial structures are inclusions of proliferation from either uterine mucosa or peritoneal serosa. The fact that the mucosa takes on decidual changes, Meyer holds, does not controvert the theory, since the decidual reaction is no longer held characteristic only of müllerian tissue. It occurs in inflammatory processes of omentum, appendix, and retroperitoneal tissue in the culdesac.

Sampson [23] has recently developed a theory which explains more simply the origin of ectopic adenomyoma. He has developed it from a remarkable series of histologic studies. He sees the tumors as results of implantation and transplantation of epithelium rather than of metaplasia.

Sampson believes that ectopic adenomyoma arise from epithelial cells which escape from the abdominal end of the open fallopian tubes during the menstrual process and which become embedded subsequently upon the pelvic peritoneum, either as a primary process or after the tissue has developed in the ovary which acts as an intermediate host. In marked contrast to Meyer, who saw the tumor as an inflammatory reaction subsequently invaded by epithelium, Sampson sees the tumor as a proliferation of epithelium, so irritating to the contiguous structures that an inflammation develops about it as a protective reaction. The theory is obtaining wide acceptance.

Sampson's work developed from a study of hemorrhagic cysts of the ovary, a condition found in 10 per cent of women between the ages of 30 and the menopause whom he operated by the abdominal route for the relief of pelvic pain. The cysts are usually bilateral and small, measuring from 2 to 4 cm. in diameter. The ovaries are adherent, and when freed, a chocolate-colored fluid escapes which is characteristic of the condition. Sampson was early struck by the marked relationship between these chocolate cysts and adenomyoma. His study soon suggested that epithelial cells escaping from the fimbriated ends of the tube during menstruation became adherent upon the contiguous ovary, and maintained the ability to proliferate. When the ovarian follicle developed and burst, the cyst cavity was invaded by these proliferating epithelial cells which soon formed a lining. A section taken from the depth of the hematoma usually showed lutein cells; the cyst from the perforation is more or less completely relined by the endometrial implants which develop on the surface of the ovary. This epithelium retains both its former structure and function. It forms structures resembling uterine glands; stroma soon appears, resembling that of the endometrium, lying between the epithelium and the ovarian tissue. The stroma varies in thickness, is usually vascular and may be thin or almost lacking. The gland spaces frequently contain old or recent blood, exactly resembling the hematomas in adenomyoma of the uterus believed to be retained menstrual blood. The histological findings varied in different specimens and in different portions of the tumor. They correspond to the cellular picture seen in the various phases of the menstrual cycle.

Exact counterparts of the epithelial structures seen in these ovarian hematomas can be found in other parts of the pelvis. They often look more like normal endometrium than do the structures seen in the ovary. Histological study shows that the hemorrhage is periodic and into closed cysts or pockets, just as occurs in the uterine hematoma of uterine adenomyoma. Sampson believes that the epithelial cells or their secretion are highly irritating to the peritoneum and that they quickly form adhesions. The ovary invaded by these cysts usually is densely adherent and chocolate colored. Dark blood may escape from the adhesions as the ovary is freed. Microscopic adenomyoma of the endothelial type occur in the adhesions. Sampson believes that many times in the life of the ovary, displaced epithelial tissue escapes into the peritoneal cavity after rupture of the follicle, and gravitates to some pocket in the folds of the pelvis. The resultant mass may remain small and quiescent or become invasive. Thus, it may cause adenomyoma by invading the uterine wall or adenomyoma of the round ligament if this structure is attacked, or adenomyoma of the sigmoid colon, etc. There is discussion as to just how the contents of the chocolate cyst stimulates the development of adenomyoma. The disease seems to spread as do implantations of ovarian papilloma, or carcinoma, on the peritoneal surface of the pelvis after rupture of the primary ovarian tumor. While Sampson insists that the chocolate cysts of the ovary are often the first step in the production of ectopic pelvic adenomyoma, he does not claim that it is the only method of production. Thus, it is possible theoretically for the epithelium escaping from the tube during menstruation to become transplanted directly upon the pelvic peritoneum and, as a result of proliferation, produce adenomyoma of the rectovaginal septum.

There has been no change in the treatment of ectopic adenomyoma since the appearance of the text. A number of observers record their experience with radium. In some cases, as in that of Herly,[24] the growth developed again after a quiescent period. The adenomyoma of the rectovaginal septum may remain long dormant. We have a case under observation where it has been quiescent for five years after hysterectomy. There are several new reported cases of adenocarcinoma in adenomyoma of the rectovaginal septum.

## FIBROIDS

**Fibroids and Sterility.**—It has long been known that fibroids are often seen in sterile women. In the 3617 fibroid cases which Lynch collected from the literature in 1913, 31.5 per cent were sterile. In his individual series of 215 fibroids in women married three or more years, 31.8 per cent were sterile. A similar compilation showed that sterility in married women in general ranged somewhere between 8 per cent and 15 per cent. That is to say, there is more than twice as much sterility in fibroid cases as in married women in general.

There are three ways to explain the relation between fibroids and sterility: (1) The fibroid causes sterility; (2) sterility causes or at least favors the fibroid; or (3) there is a common factor which favors both the fibroid and sterility.

1. Does the fibroid cause sterility? There are many statistics in the literature tending to prove that the fibroid causes sterility by reason of its presence, and that the larger the tumor, the more likely is sterility. The statistics of Schorler, Young, and Williams, and Goetze may be rearranged to support this view. In Goetze's series, the percentage of sterility ranged from 13.6 per cent in cases in which the fibroid was the size of an apple to 50 per cent in cases with growths the size of a man's head or bigger. The larger tumors may favor sterility by causing disturbances in the uterine circulation which create discharges which lesson the likelihood of conception, or, by changes in the endometrium, interfere with the embedding of the egg. Yet pregnancy is often seen in the presence of very large tumors. Nearly any physician of experience can recall pregnancies associated with fibroids the size of four, five, or even six months pregnancy. In fact, pregnancies with fibroids are common enough to have created a considerable literature. They are rarely seen with submucous fibroids in which hemorrhage is a predominant symptom. In this connection, one should recall that pregnancy occasionally occurs in other conditions associated with marked leukorrhea. It may occur with carcinoma of the cervix, even when leukorrhea and bleeding have been symptoms.

It, therefore, appears that fibroids often cause sterility. Yet, in this discussion we must recall that fibroids usually develop comparatively late in a woman's menstrual life whereas marriage and pregnancy ordinarily occur early. Between marriage and the time when the fibroid has attained a size or created conditions favoring sterility, the woman might have had many children, unless there was some other factor which was responsible for sterility.

This view is supported by the fact that nearly all women who have submucous fibroids have borne children. Goetze found that 91 per cent of his submucous fibroids had had children. Eighty per cent of the submucous cases of our own series were also parous. The submucous fibroid usually originates in the puerperium, being the result of a displacement of the interstitial growth during retraction and involution of the uterus after labor.

The above indicates that sterility from fibroids may be due only to changes resulting from the position of the tumor, the presence of leukorrheal or sanguinous discharges, or because of circulatory or degenerative changes in the tumor. In an individual series of 215 fibroid cases of women married three years or more, Lynch [25] found that only 169 had been pregnant, a sterility of 31.8 per cent. It seems difficult to believe that the tumor *per se* was responsible for the sterility in this series because the growths, for the most part, were only a few centimeters in size. Even in Goetze's series of large tumors, sterility was present in only 50 per cent.

2. Does sterility cause fibroids? The affirmative of this question has been argued for years, ever since Stephen Bayle, in 1807, wrote on the

question. In this discussion, we should divide our cases into virgins and non-virgins. It is argued that fibroids are common in virgins, because the uterus has been denied its opportunity to hypertrophy in its physiologic manner, *i.e.*, pregnancy. This view was advanced by Bayle and has received warm support from many men who do surgery of the celibate woman of religious orders in whom fibroids are undoubtedly common. The view is interesting but does not yet admit of proof since there are no large series of accurate observations concerning the pelvic organs of virgin women. It may be urged with equal right that there are unduly large proportions of women with underdeveloped rather than overdeveloped pelvic organs in the religious orders and that fibroids are frequent in uteri that are immature. More is known concerning the frequency of fibroids in married women who seek relief for sterility. The results of tubal inflammation is the common cause of sterility. If sterility *per se* favored fibroid development, we should see many fibroids associated with old inflammatory disease of pyogenic origin. Yet the fibroid incidence is not great in these conditions.

3. There is a common factor favoring both sterility and fibroid development. In a study of uterine retroversions and retroflexions following delivery, Lynch found that the women who had had posterior uterine displacements of congenital origin were less likely to become pregnant than those whose uterus was in normal position prior to pregnancy, suggesting that the sterility in retrodisplacements is largely due to congenital causes. Study of sterility and fibroids also strongly suggests that sterility long antedated the fibroid. Data from the retroflexion studies suggests that there is a common origin for both the sterility and the fibroid. In this connection, it is worth while to recall that Bayle, in 1807, wrote that fibroids, while common in virgins, were also frequently found in married women who were sterile. The first part of the statement alone seems to have made an impression on the literature. We believe that the literature warrants the belief that both fibroids and sterility (in the absence of known causes) are due to some congenital condition expressing itself clinically as lack of uterine development.

**Pregnancy after Radiation.**—It has long been known that pregnancy following radiation was likely to result in monstrosities. This view dates to 1903 when Bohn described deformities in frogs resulting from radiation of the embryos. Gilman and Baetjer in the same year reported their observations from raying fertilized ova of amblystoma. They found a characteristic deformity in the head and brain. Hartwig in more recent time has done a tremendous amount of work along these lines, making observations after raying spermatozoa, non-impregnated ova and impregnated ova. He worked with the semen of frogs, the eggs of seagulls and of a number of nematodes. Since then Baldwin, Bagg, Little and Bagg, and a great number of others have worked with experimental animals, and described deformities resulting from radiation, the most common being in the eyes and brain. The observations of Lacassagne and Coutard, in

1923, are of considerable interest. These observers found that the progeny of female rabbits that had been previously radiated were less resistant than normal in that there was more "infant mortality" in the cases that had been radiated than in the normal controls. Arrested development was also frequently noted in the embryos found in the tubes at time of autopsy. Others have shown that the same distressing results were likely to follow no matter whether the female animal was rayed before fertilization or during pregnancy.

The literature affords abundant evidence that the fibroid should not be treated with radium or Roentgen ray during pregnancy, although there are a number of cases reported in which the fetus has shown little or no injury. Yet the literature offers no criterion as to what dose can be safely borne during pregnancy without resultant fetal injury. The fact that there are deformities is positive and should be carefully considered. Aschenheim, in 1920, reported a case in which treatment had been given between the second and sixth months of gestation. The child was premature at eight months, was microcephalic, had deficiencies of sight and was an imbecile. Stettner, in 1921, reported a fibroid that had been treated with Roentgen ray when the woman was two months pregnant, the condition not being known. An underdeveloped child was born at eight months with hypospadius, strabismus, neuroretinitis, and definite mental changes. The child could not speak at two years of age. Aschenheim's case was treated with rays evidently of the short wave type, while Stettner's case was probably of the deep therapy type, the dosage being considerable in each. Lawson,[26] in 1925, reports the Roentgen ray treatment of a fibroid in a woman pregnant four months. The child was delivered by a cesarean section somewhat before term, and remained mentally and physically backward for two years before developing normally. On the contrary, there are several reported cases where women during pregnancy were treated with radium for uterine or vaginal cancers without causing known deformity in the child. Such cases have been reported by Berkeley in 1921, Field in 1922, and Bailey and Bagg, two cases in 1923. The method, however, cannot be considered safe.

There is also some literature concerning pregnancy following some time after pelvic radiation. Werner,[27] in 1921, showed that radiation of the pelves of adult women does not necessarily inhibit the power of conception, predispose to abortion or premature labor, disturb parturition, or cause monstrosities. He studied 24 cases that were known to have followed a series of 1542 cases that had been radiated for benign hemorrhages, 552 of which were fibroids. Thirteen cases came to term with normal living children, nine aborted, one child was born four weeks premature, one pregnancy was terminated by the removal of a fibroid uterus which had started to grow again. Stacy,[28] in 1922, reviewed the pregnancies that were known to have followed cases that were radiated in the Mayo Clinic. The total number of women who had been radiated at time of her report was 1013. Pregnancy was known to have followed in ten cases; four of the children were normal and born at term, three were stillborn, two cases aborted, and the tenth had not been delivered when the article was written. Clark and Keene reported their experience in 1922. They had radiated 527 cases. Seven women were known to have become subsequently pregnant. Only two of these were delivered at term of normal children. Steiger reports a case of pregnancy following a two-year period of amenorrhea. A normal child was born at term. Bailey and Bagg report two cases where women radiated during pregnancy in regions other than the pelvis were also delivered of deformed children. They also report two cases in which pregnancy followed radiation for fibroids. The first became pregnant nine months after treatment, and was delivered at term of a large stillborn child; the second became pregnant one and a half years after treatment and was delivered of a normal child at term. Pemberton, in *Surgery, Gynecology and Obstetrics,* in August 1924, reported four pregnancies following some time after rather light redium treatments given by Graves in Boston. There was no deformity of the fetus. While these case reports present no complications other than stillbirths and abortions, Naujoks,[29] in December, 1923, reported a case in which there is clear proof of injury to the fetus because of radiation of the ovary before pregnancy. The dosage, however, was large.

**Occurrence of Malignancy with Fibroids.**—Essen-Moeller,[30] in 1921, reported malignancy in 22 of 700 fibroid cases, six cancers and 16 sarcoma. Mayo, in 1922, recorded that 4 per cent of his fibroids presented some evidence of malignancy. Vogt,[31] in 1923, in 1216 fibroids in the University of Pennsylvania found 30 sarcoma. Eight of these could be traced directly to changes of the fibroid, 0.6 per cent. Ten sarcoma were early, 12 were moderately advanced, and eight presented extensive involvement. That sarcoma is a dangerous condition is well shown by the results. Twenty-four had radical operation. There was a follow up of 16 cases with only two cures and 14 fatalities. Masson,[32] in 1923, reported sarcomatous changes in 44 of 4322 fibroid cases in the Mayo clinic (1 per cent). Apparent cure was obtained in only 36 cases. Aschoff, in the same year, found that one per cent of the fibroids in the Freiburg Clinic had sarcomatous change. Reed and Charlton,[33] in 1923, reported 11 uterine sarcoma of which nine developed in fibroids. Truesdale, in 1923, found six malignancies in 300 fibroids. Jeff Miller,[34] in 1924, reported four malignancies in 127 fibroids operated in New Orleans; three were carcinoma of the cervix and one fibrosarcoma. The Pennsylvania State Cancer Commission[35] in their 1924 report show that in 45 cancers of the uterine body, fibroids had been present before the malignancy in seven cases.

**Treatment of Fibroids.**—There have been many articles on fibroids in the literature of the last few years dealing for the most part with therapy. The great majority emphasize that we have at our disposal three great therapeutic agents, the modern Roentgen ray, radium, and surgery, each of which has definite advantages and disadvantages. While the literature is largely composed of articles advocating one method to the exclusion of the others, there is no doubt that the truly conservative man will utilize all three.

As has been urged in the text, the treatment of fibroids should be divided into four headings, expectant treatment, Roentgen ray, radium, and operation.

*Expectant Treatment.*—The opinion is gaining ground, fortunately, that too many fibroids are subjected to treatment, and that a very large proportion of these tumors are relatively harmless. Lockyer concludes that 55 per cent give rise to no symptoms. There is little doubt that many small fibroids are actively treated largely because the practitioners are misled by the literature as to the frequency of complications from fibroid tumors. We have frequently urged that the fibroid literature in texts has been compiled from study of large tumors. The statistics of Noble, Deaver, and others, which expressed the condition of older times no longer represent the frequency of serious complications in fibroids seen at the present time. Some indeed, as William Neil, Jr., in 1924, urge that uncomplicated tumors, even the size of a five months pregnancy, be let alone if they are not giving symptoms. The existence of a fibroid heart is again disputed by Winter.

The view of Neil represents the extreme and does not appear to us as a safe procedure unless the woman is near the menopause and the physicians at her disposal are comparatively unskilled in surgery, and especially not versed in gynecologic conditions. We have elsewhere alluded to the danger attending the use of emergency surgical methods in conditions which are chronic and not immediately threatening life. Personally, we believe that any woman had better keep a tumor not yet giving symptoms even if it is the size of a five months pregnancy rather than be filled with a mass of intestinal adhesions resulting from an unskilful surgical operation, if she recovered. Nor is it safe to allow a tumor of such size to go untreated. Fibroids of much smaller size develop serious degenerations. Moreover, they may grow quickly. Recently we have seen a tumor in three years develop from the size of a large hickory nut to several masses larger than a man's fist, and compel operations because of degenerations. We are of the opinion that growing fibroids, even 4 or 5 cm. in diameter, may be treated in young women early by myomectomy rather than allowing them to grow to a size requiring hysterectomy.

There is no doubt but that fibroid tumors presenting symptoms represent serious conditions. Yearly we operate many cases which have bled so long that they cannot be safely operated without repeated blood transfusions. While deaths in untreated cases are seldom seen in the literature at the present time, Dartigues,[36] in 1923, is not alone in calling attention to the frequency of serious complications.

*Roentgen Ray.*—During the last few years, there has been a tremendous improvement in Roentgen ray therapy. This is due in large part to the employment of rays of shorter wave length than formerly used. The wave length of these rays approximates those of radium. The newer tubes permit high voltage (200,000 to 280,000) delivered at the Roentgen ray terminal. Proper screening will eliminate the rays of long wave length (which do not penetrate deeply), and permit the raying of the deeper tissues with homogeneous rays which pass through the body tissues in a straight line with a negligible amount of reflection or refraction from contact with body cells.

Even before the improvements, striking results were frequently obtained in the treatment of fibroids whose chief symptom was hemorrhage. The defects of the older methods were their uncertainty and the number of burns which ensued. With the improved machines, the results are better in that amenorrhea can be produced in nearly all cases. The development of roentgenology has taken away treatment with the newer machines from the hands of the general practitioner since the rays are extremely powerful and capable of much harm, if unskilfully applied. This will probably diminish the number of burns. Yet there are other dangers. One must be extremely careful as to what tissues are radiated. Smithies, in 1924, reported a case dying from injury of the adrenals and Whipple has shown the frequency of intestinal burns.

The great defect of the treatment with fibroids is that results depend upon the induction of a menopause by the destruction of the ovarian follicles. Some claim that there is also a direct effect upon the tumor but it is a fact that little or nothing can be accomplished without producing amenorrhea. The treatment, therefore, is not adapted to persons in whom the retention of ovarian activity is desirable, which in our minds restricts it nearly completely to women about to enter the menopause. Roentgen ray treatment of fibroids probably has a little wider field of usefulness than does radium since it may be given to large tumors, to cases with old pelvic inflammatory disease of the adnexa and to submucous tumors without necessarily producing harm. Whether it accomplished much in these cases is still an open question. Seitz [37] and Wintz,[38] who are enthusiastic advocates of the method, claim it is the best treatment in cases where sarcoma is suspected in the fibroid mass, in which case they give doubly strong doses. Many others disagree. It is evident, of course, that in case there are benign degenerations of the fibroid, that Roentgen ray cannot cure, and that the logical treatment is surgical removal of the mass. It also would appear that if the rays did act upon the fibroid tissue to any considerable extent that Roentgen ray given to tumors with degenerations or submucous growths would be productive of harm exactly as occurs in radium. The treatment should not be given without preliminary curettage to exclude the chance of malignancy since adenocarcinoma of the fundus is not best treated with any method of radiation, although there is less agreement as to sarcoma. The seriousness of the modern method of Roentgen ray treatment demands that the case be under the general direction of a gynecologist and not in that of the roentgenologist.

There is a long list of case reports in the literature of the last two or three years. Béclère,[39] in 1921, reported 300 cases treated with Roentgen ray. He claimed the reduction of the size of the tumor was so constant that an abdominal tumor diagnosed as uterine fibroid which does not shrink after Roentgen ray cannot be considered to be fibroid. The authors are not able to corroborate this opinion from their review of the literature. Gal, Krönig, and Gauss, in 1921, also strongly urged the wider employment of the Roentgen ray and feel that marked menorrhagia does not contraindicate it. Essen-Moeller, in 1924, reported 103 fibroids treated by Roentgen ray, 32 of which were big enough to show above the superior strait. Fifty cases returned to normal size, ten were reduced but not markedly, in 20 there was no change. Twenty-three were lost in the follow-up. Martindale, and Hanks,[40] in 1924, reported their results, the latter in a series of 100 cases. She prefers this therapy because in her judgment it is easier and safer than radium. She claims that it reduces large tumors more certainly and works more slowly, sometimes taking two or three months before the menopause is established, which gives the individual time for readjustment to meet the distressing condition. The latter point has not been noticed by us, since we find that hot flashes constitute an early complaint after the first treatment. Menopausal symptoms came on in ten days with Pirazzoli's two large tumors recorded in December, 1924. Gellhorn, in 1921, reviewed the literature and collected 2982 fibroid cases treated with Roentgen rays, with 95.6 per cent symptomatic cures and 4.4 per cent failures. Better results have been obtained in single series. Gauss, and Friedrich had 98.4 per cent cures and 1.6 per cent failures in 425 cases treated with Roentgen ray. Gellhorn, however, feels that in selected cases radium is safer than the Roentgen ray.

Not all the reports are favorable, however, to this method of therapy. Nor would they be if the results accomplished are due to the destruction of ovarian function, a subject we reviewed in the text. Hempel-Jörgensen,[41] in 1924, reviews five cases, all of which were treated unsuccessfully with the modern Roentgen ray. One case had had radium in addition. The tumors were submucous in three instances and intramural and subserous in the others. All came to operation. Hempel-Jörgensen reviews the list of men who advocated the Roentgen ray for submucous fibroids at that time, finding that Doederlein, Krönig, and others advocated it. Lundquist,[42] in 1922, reported a small series in which he contrasted the results obtained in modern Roentgen ray and radium. Thirty-four cases were treated with Roentgen ray. Amenorrhea was produced in 22, seven cases were improved, and the treatment was unsuccessful in one. Forty-eight cases were treated with intrauterine radium. Amenorrhea was produced in 26, improvement was noted in seven, and the treatment was unsuccessful in 15. Radium was applied vaginally only in 12 cases. Amenorrhea was produced in five, the condition was improved in six, and one was not improved. The tumors were reduced in size in between 75 per cent and 80 per cent of each series.

The question of dosage is of the greatest interest. The subject, however, is too complicated to be considered here, as it goes a long way into the realms of physics. The student, therefore, is referred to the modern bibliography of the Roentgen ray. There are, however, different ideas concerning dosage held by roentgenologists of different nationalities. The Germans still favor, as they did years ago, massive doses, believing that the reduction of the fibroid depends entirely upon castration and that this result is produced more certainly by one large dose. The French, on the other hand, believe in divided doses, which are given usually at weekly intervals. Some of the French authors feel that these also act upon the tumor and sterilize the follicular apparatus of the ovary just as effectively as if the massive dose were used. They claim that divided doses minimize the shock to the patient and prevent the reactions seen after a single heavy dose, even in the German clinics.

Evidence that the divided dosage is reasonable was adduced by Warren and Whipple,[43] in 1923. These investigators approached the question through animal experimentation. They found that the maximum sublethal dose applied to the abdomen caused the same amount of destruction in the animal's intestines no matter whether it is given in single doses, or in smaller doses if repeated within six-day intervals. On the other hand, they found that frequently doses given six days or more apart gave no evidence of summation. On the contrary, there was a suggestion that the tissues may have become more tolerant.

*Radium.*—Many have recorded their experiences with radium during the last two years and there is more agreement as to its indications and limitations. Keene,[44] writing in 1924, stated that it is not applicable to more than 50 per cent of cases and feels that it has definite contraindications. While these are in essence identical with the text, we shall again give them. Radium should not be used in: (1) tumors larger than a three months' pregnancy; (2) rapidly growing tumors, for fear of sarcomatous change or preëxisting benign degenerations; (3) uncomplicated tumors of any size giving rise to symptoms other than abnormal menstruation; (4) tumors associated with pelvic pain; (5) pedunculated tumors of any type; (6) tumors producing hemorrhage and complicated by demonstrable adnexal pathology; (7) when the bleeding from the tumor is not sufficient to explain a marked secondary anemia; (8) tumors in young women; (9) tumors so distorting the uterine cavity that the radium cannot be introduced well above the internal os; (10) in cases where the differentiation between fibroid and adnexal tumor cannot be definitely determined; (11) fibroids or myofibropathic hemorrhage in nervous women; (12) in cases of radiophobia. Nearly all agree with these postulates. Many have had bad experiences after radiating fibroid cases associated with unexplained anemias resulting from the absorption of toxic substances from degenerative areas. Nearly all agree that radium is not applicable for the routine treatment of submucous tumors.

Burnam[45] has treated successfully a number of comparatively large fibroids with radium, 30 of the tumors ranging between the size of a four and seven months' pregnancy. He has used large doses of radium, which prohibits his method from universal adoption. Burnam feels that as far as bleeding is concerned radium is just as effectual in large tumors as in the smaller growths, although larger doses are required than in the smaller tumors. He uses at one time an intrauterine carrier containing an emanation equivalent of 1½ Gm. of radium. By moving the carrier, he treats all areas of the uterine cavity and thus limits the chance of an excessive dose for any one place. He has given as much as 3 gram-hours radiation in the uterine cavity without bad effects. This treatment is augmented by radiating the pelvis through lateral portals over either ovary for a dosage of 10 gram-hours, which he believes has almost the same effect as the 1500 mc.-hour intrauterine treatment. The radium is held a distance of three inches from the skin. External radiation in addition to the intrauterine treatment appears to him as indispensable for large fibroids with short uterine cavities. The treatment requires about five hours for the full 20 gram-hour external dosage and should be done at two or more sittings. This is in contrast to the treatment of smaller growths in which the standard intrauterine dose to produce permanent amenorrhea has been 1½ gram-hours, giving an amenorrhea of at least a year in nearly all cases and a permanent amenorrhea in about 80 per cent of cases. Burnam urges that each operator determine for himself what dosage is necessary for the treatment of his individual case since it is impossible to interpret the intrauterine dosage on a gram-hour basis independent of the amount of radium used and the time consumed. In his 30 cases, Burnam found that the uterus returned to normal size in 15, to the size of a six weeks' pregnancy in four, and did not grow again in any of the 19 cases. In 11, the reduction in size was unsatisfactory, although there was relief of symptoms.

Ward,[46] up to 1924, also had treated successfully 17 cases larger than a four months' pregnancy. He had 14 satisfactory follow-ups. Eleven tumors were reduced in size, many to nearly normal. He had used comparatively small amounts of radium, giving from 1200 to 3600 Mgm.-hours. Contraindications to operation were present in all cases. Two of the cases had submucous growths and developed toxic absorption and finally sloughed considerable tissues. Although both recovered, the convalescence was attended by temperature and one case remained 30 days in the hospital, the other 79 on account of the sloughing mass.

Bailey,[47] whose work with radium in gynecology is well known, does not care to treat fibroids greater than the size of a three months' pregnancy with radium. He has had nine large tumors up to 1924, five of which extended above navel. Of these five, one was lost in the follow-up and possibly had a hysterectomy at another hospital. He was compelled to do hysterectomies on the other four. The tumor of one was very edematous and larger than when he first saw it. Another was much smaller but was filled with degeneration areas. We have had one case larger than a four months' pregnancy in which the symptom of profuse bleeding was arrested and the tumor itself returned to the size of a six weeks' pregnancy in about six months. A disagreeable menopause was the only complication.

Faure[48] used comparatively small doses of radium, repeating the treatment if the results were unsatisfactory. Writing in 1921, he preferred radium but admitted that with improved Roentgen ray machines the latter might be preferred. Clark, Lundquist and others emphasized the fact that radium in selected cases gives excellent results.

Personally we do not see a great field for the radium treatment of fibroids. Theoretically the treatment is logical but there are too many contraindications. Practically, the treatment is applicable to certain small tumors in which hemorrhage is the cardinal symptom. Since radium acts chiefly upon the tumor and more slightly upon the ovary, this treatment is more logical than is the Roentgen ray if we agree that the retention of ovarian function is advisable. Practically, however, it is nearly impossible to treat the tumor successfully without affecting the ovaries. When comparatively small doses of radium have been given in the uterine cavity, the endometrium generally atrophies and no longer responds to the stimulation of the ovary. Endarteritis causes an occlusion of many smaller vessels and there is a change from myomatous to fibrous tissue resulting in shrinkage of the tumor and restriction of the bleeding. The theoretical advantage of radium over Roentgen ray is less marked if the tumor is large, since the feeling is crystallizing that destruction of ovarian follicle is necessary to ensure the marked reduction in the size of the tumor. Therefore, in large tumors, intrauterine radiation should be supplemented by cross-fire through the abdomen with either Roentgen ray or radium. Practically the treatment of the smaller tumors is likely to cause permanent amenorrhea. Whether the future will prove that radiation of the pituitary gland will cause shrinkage of the fibroid tumor remains to be proved. The subject is under investigation.

The limitations of the treatment are real, and demand complete recognition. They concern both age of patient and condition of the tumor. There exists, morever, a certain danger. The restrictions of age are based only upon the destruction of ovarian tissue and the precipitation of the menopause. For that reason, it is best suited for cases approaching the menopause and is not desirable for young women.

The fact that it will not cure submucous tumors demands careful consideration since growths of this type constitute a large proportion of the fibroids causing symptoms. Moreover, it is not always easy to diagnose submucous tumors prior to removal. We have radiated several tumors of three months' pregnancy size or more in which it was finally found that in each case the hemorrhage was dependent upon a submucous tumor not larger than 4 or 5 cm. in diameter. All of these cases had been practically exsanguinated and were not good risks for operation. Radiation gave no results. After nearly three months' wait, during which time patients had been repeatedly transfused, all finally came to operation. The frequency of degeneration in large tumors is well known. The larger the tumor, therefore, the more likely you are to encounter complications from absorption of toxic products resulting from degenerations. The treatment is not without danger because of the chance of lighting up a previous, but unsuspected, inflammation. One case of ours with a large tumor, the size of a five months' pregnancy, a bad risk for operation, was hospitalized for more than three months from a peritonitis resulting from such a reaction. We had carefully examined her previously and had not been able to detect any sign of an old inflammation since she was fat and not easy to examine. Moreover, we have had a number of cases radiated by us develop extremely severe menopausal symptoms, and feel in consequence it is not a method well adapted for the treatment of nervous women.

There is no doubt but that atresia of the uterine canal has been a common sequel to intrauterine radiation. The stricture is often followed by pyometra.

*Operation.*—This method of therapy should be considered in two sections, hysterectomy and myomectomy.

HYSTERECTOMY.—From the practical standpoint of cure, hysterectomy far surpasses Roentgen ray or radium since with the removal of the entire uterus and tumor goes all fear of subsequent malignancy. The shortcomings of the method are that it is destructive. Moreover, there is risk of life, definite though small; much pain as a direct result of operation followed by a certain amount of semi-invalidism; and considerable monetary expense. Yet there is a broad field for hysterectomy and one which is undoubtedly permanent, in cases which are not suitable for radium or Roentgen ray, or where these measures have failed because the tumor has caused pressure or has degenerated and caused pain, or where malignancy, or marked inflammatory disease, or adenomyoma are complications. The uterus and tumor are usually removed by supravaginal hysterectomy. The one weak point of this procedure is that cancer may later supervene in a cervix which has been allowed to remain. Scattered case reports constantly appear in the literature. In 268 cervical cancer cases cited by the Pennsylvania State Cancer Commission, in 1924,[35] there were nine which developed in the cervix after supravaginal hysterectomy for fibroids. This suggests a need for panhysterectomy which we feel should be done wherever practical. In case it is not deemed wise, the cervix, if diseased, should be cored out from above if it has not been previously repaired just before the laparotomy. In our own experience, the mortality of panhysterectomy and supravaginal hysterectomy are practically identical. A hysterectomy seems ideal in that the surgeon may leave the ovaries while removing the tumor mass and uterus. Occasionally, however, the ovaries later may become cystic because of disturbance of the ovarian circulation. The literature abounds in descriptions of methods which claim to permit removal of the uterus without interfering with the ovarian circulation. They fail since it is impossible to maintain the integrity of the utero-ovarian branches of the ovarian circulation after removal of the uterus. Fortunately, it makes comparatively little difference in the great mass of cases.

MYOMECTOMY.—There is no doubt that myomectomy is increasing in popularity. The procedure is ideal in that it removes the offending structures, and disturbs the pelvic organs to a minimum degree. In our opinion, it is the treatment of the future. Yet at present it cannot be applied to all cases in active menstrual life since the tumors are often so large that myomectomy cannot be safely done. Moreover, it is not the operation of choice for men beginning surgery.

In the past, myomectomy has not been popular because the mortality as given in the text is higher than that of hysterectomy. We have many times emphasized that mortalities reported in surgical texts usually belong to an older era, and do not represent results in good hands at the present time. The proper technic of myomectomy involves much detail. It should be done by a technic evolved for the surgical treatment of chronic conditions and not that of emergency procedures. If the patient is left with large knots and rough surfaces placed to invite intestinal adhesions, the performance of myomectomy is a serious error. Roentgen ray or radium, or even supravaginal hysterectomy, would be more rational procedures.

When one has developed a proper technic for myomectomy, an enormous mass of tumor structures can be safely enucleated. The authors are much impressed with the frequent seriousness of menopausal symptoms, both following radiation and operation, and feel that in myomectomy there is a way of avoiding this distressing complication. By operating tumors which have begun to grow rapidly after considerable observation, myomectomy will come to prevent more radical measures.

Myomectomy may be used occasionally even in the face of hemorrhage since the results indicate that the bleeding in fibroids is not chiefly dependent upon ovarian activity. Recent confirmation of this belief was given by Schmid's [49] report, in 1923, of the follow-up of 88 myomectomies in the Prague Clinic. In case of doubt, the uterine cavity should be opened and carefully inspected before a definite type of operation is decided upon. The presence of pyometra contraindicates myomectomy. In our opinion, myomectomy can be safely extended to women of 38 to 40 after exclusion of all evidence of malignancy, provided the uterine tissue permits good closure. We urge this because of the belief that an artificial menopause is a distinctly pathological situation. Ott, in 1924, among others asks why surgery should be delayed until the case is in a serious condition. Mayo, in 1922, reported 504 myomectomies with a mortality of 0.8 per cent. Giles, in the same year, advocates myomectomies up to the fortieth year. Bonney, in 1922, reported 100 cases with the removal of from one to thirty fibroids. If menorrhagia were the complaint, he opened the uterus to be sure all masses were removed. His complications consisted almost entirely of hemorrhage. There were two deaths, one from shock and one from hemorrhage. Five of the cases subsequently went through pregnancy.

Theoretically, the operation permits of subsequent conception, although care must be exhibited with each individual case. Gouillioud,[50] in 1924, reported 95 cases in which pregnancy occurred 125 times following myomectomy. One hundred went to term and resulted in living children. The series was marred by uterine rupture in three instances, one of which was fatal. This, in our judgment, is not necessarily an indictment against myomectomy, since we believe that all will come to agree that the closure in myomectomies presents the same problems as does that in cesareans, and that pregnancies following extensive myomectomy should be delivered by cesarean section before the onset of labor. There are, in addition to Gouilloud's report a number of other small series of pregnancies following myomectomy recorded in the French literature.

## MALIGNANT TUMORS OF THE UTERUS

**Carcinoma of the Uterus.**—*Etiology.*—The infection has received decided support through the work of Nuzum,[51] who in 1924 reported to the American Clinical Congress of Surgeons his studies of several years' duration. From inoculation of dextrose acitic fluid with fragments of an early carcinoma removed from the human breast, Nuzum has grown anaërobically a filterable micrococcus which, when introduced into white mice and dogs, causes an epithelial tumor resembling carcinoma and which gives off metastases. From these tumors in the experimental animals, the same organism was obtained by inoculating dextrose acitic fluid. The organism was injected into the leg of a man of 70, who apparently had been sensitized to carcinoma by having a cancer of the face. A tumor mass resulted which, when removed, gave the structure of an epithelioid cancer. The paper was printed in 1925. This work, although strikingly suggestive to the very highest degree, cannot be accepted as proof positive until it has been presented in complete form and has been confirmed by other independent investigators. We have stressed in the textbook the importance which we attach to heredity as one of the etiologic factors in cancer and have urged that the importance of heredity is not generally appreciated chiefly because family histories are not well taken in the usual hospital record. In our clinic, we carefully distinguish between patients in whom the family history is well known and those in whom it is not known. We do not count as family history any record in which the patient is not familiar with the causes of death of mother, father, grandparents, and some of the collaterals. We have been struck in our cases with the very high percentage of cancer in the family of cases in our series in which such data were known.

Little,[52] in 1923, also discussed the question from records in the Eugenic Record office of the Carnegie Institution. This material had been furnished by persons of intelligence, conscientiously endeavoring to provide accurate family histories for scientific purposes. His study showed that cancer occurs much more frequently in those in whom there is a family cancerous history than is to be expected from the general cancer mortality figures.

Writing in 1923, Gideon Wells[53] discussed the influence of heredity on the occurrence of cancer. Wells urged that "statistical evidence in literature of the present time may be dismissed with the statement that in the question of human cancer heredity, all existing statistical evidence is valueless for any exact information on this subject and must remain so until such time as we have necropsy records on all persons dying in several generations." He stated that "in considering the relationship of heredity to cancer even a single error in diagnosis might totally destroy the value of an entire family history making it appear that cancer was present in a branch of a family when it was not, or that it had failed to appear in a certain branch in which it actually did exist." No student of carcinoma can deny the truth of these remarks. This being the case, it seems reasonable to believe that scientific data on the subject will never be obtainable in humans for many, many generations, in fact, until the time when all who die shall be autopsied and studied by skilled pathologists.

Yet in the meantime, there is the greatest need of impressing the medical profession with the fact that early carcinoma alone is curable and its diagnosis in that stage is often a very difficult matter. Anything that focuses the mind of the practitioner upon the diagnosis of early cancer should be of value. There is, we believe, strongly suggestive evidence which, while not qualifying as scientific proof, is quite enough to convince any thoughtful practitioner of medicine that descendants of cancerous patients or persons with cancerous relatives should be viewed medically as more likely to have cancer than those in whom there is no family history. Sickness from cancer which causes death is rarely confused with any other disease and makes an impression upon others of the family which is passed on to several generations following, provided always that the individual knows the family. This view, of course, does not permit consideration of the fact that many individuals, while having cancer, die from some other disease before cancer gives sufficient clinical manifestations to call attention to its presence.

*Classification of Uterine Cancer, According to Histology.*—Following along the general lines established by Broders,[54] in "Cancer of the Lip," Martzloff,[55] in 1923, reported histological and clinical study of 387 cancers of the uterus seen in the Johns Hopkins Gynecologic Department prior to 1920. The object of this study was to determine whether there was a definite relation between the histomorphology of the predominant cancer cells and the degree of clinical malignancy. The material fell into three histologic groups, according as the predominant cancer cells were spinal-cell type, fat spindle, or transitional. The investigator's work showed that the tumors composed chiefly of spinal-cell forms were the least malignant, the transitional cell type were more malignant and the fat spindle-celled type were the most malignant. The adenocarcinoma fell between the spinal- and transitional-cell groups in malignancy. Martzlof's observations warrant the belief that epithelial pearls in the carcinoma are significant only when they occur in the spinal-cell group of tumors when they indicate a lessened degree of malignancy. He found that there were carcinomatous extensions from the primary tumor into the broad ligament in the first six months of the symptomatic disease in all groups except the spinal-cell type. Less than 10 per cent of the patients with broad ligament involvement lived more than one year following operation.

Pomeroy and Strauss,[56] in 1924, reported a series of cases studied along the same line. Their material consisted of 75 cases which were carefully studied. This material fell into the following groups: six cancers of the spindle-celled type with pearls; 31 spindle-celled type without pearls; 21 transitional-type tumors; six fat spindle-celled type growths and 11 adenocarcinoma. The cases which did best clinically were the spindle-celled type without pearls and the adenocarcinoma. They found, moreover, that 71 per cent of the cases in which radium gave marked palliation were transitional-celled types. Their work brings up the question as to whether the transitional-celled type cases are not very likely to respond favorably to radium.

*Radium Treatment of Cervical Cancers.*—Von Seuffert,[57] in 1922, reported Doederlein's results with mesothorium and radium in a series of 500 cervical cancers in Munich. The cases were observed between 1913 and 1916 inclusive and were contrasted with the results that were obtained with the 265 cases that were operated between 1908 and 1912 inclusive. Doederlein divided his material into two groups, one which was radiated completely and the other which left before the treatments were finished. He claimed to have cured by radium substances for a five-year period, 10 per cent of the inoperable cases, which were radiated completely; 36 per cent of the borderline cases of the same groups; as well as 80 per cent of the inoperable cancers. Less favorable results were obtained in the series which he says were incompletely radiated, although he claims a five-year cure in 20 per cent of the borderline cases and 48 per cent of the operable cases in this subdivision. Doederlein has not operated a cervical cancer since 1913. Von Seuffert contrasted the results obtained by radium with the 265 cases which had been treated by surgery, in which cure was obtained by operation in only 5 per cent of 57 borderline cases and in 46 per cent of 110 operable cases. There was injury of the adjacent tissue in 9 per cent of the cases radiated and of 10 per cent of the cases which were operated. He said that even in the cases which were not cured by radium, the duration of life was 50 per cent greater in the operable group than in the similar cases that had been treated by surgery; 45 per cent greater in the borderline cases that were radiated than those which were operated, and 55 per cent greater in the inoperable cases than in those which had been untreated prior to 1913.

Seitz,[58] in 1922, reported his five-year cures with cervical cancers that were treated by small doses of radium and the Roentgen ray. Fifty per cent of eight cervical cases and 17 per cent of 18 borderline cases were alive and free from symptoms five years after the beginning of treatment. Of the total group of 58 cases with cervical carcinoma, 12, or 20.9 per cent, are still alive. Seitz states that these figures compare favorably with those treated by the Wertheim operation, a point which we feel is quite unfair. To be of the greatest value, the comparisons on the results of surgery and radium should be made in similar groups. Seitz quoted the statistics of a number of other authors in German literature. He stated that Doederlein treated 205 cervical cancers with radium with 40 survivals for the five-year period (19.5 per cent); Bumm treated 78 cases with radium with 11 five-year survivals (14 per cent); Baisch 42 cases with seven survivals

(16 per cent); Klein 73 cases with eight survivals (12 per cent); Heymann 26 cases with seven five-year cures (26.9 per cent). Seitz believes that the excellent results obtained in his series were not due entirely to the radium but that the Roentgen ray played a very important part. Thus, there were 56 per cent of five-year cures of the patients treated predominantly by the Roentgen ray and 53 per cent of five-year cures in the cases treated exclusively with radium, percentages which are practically identical.

Beuttner,[59] in 1923, reported his five-year cures in a series of 63 cases treated by him in Geneva. Four of nine operable cases were cured as were four of eight borderline cases, and three of 25 cases in which there was a crater of the cervix and a comparatively slight infiltration of the parametrium. As a result of his study, Beuttner reached the same conclusion as did Doederlein, who stated that he could have cured by operation only about 50 per cent of the patients who appeared to have been cured for four or five years by radium.

Heymann,[60] in 1924, reported the results of 505 cervical cancers during 1914 to 1921, inclusive, in the Radiumhemmet in Stockholm. The report appears well controlled and perfectly convincing. Each case counted as a five-year cure was examined by the author five years after treatment, the cases being brought back to Stockholm for examination by a government grant. All cases dying within the five-year period were counted as due to cancer although it may be that death in two or three cases was not due to cancer. There were 217 cases available for the five-year study; 19, or 8.7 per cent, being operable and 181, or 91.3 per cent, were borderline and inoperable and were studied together, while treatment was refused to 7.5 per cent in which the growth was too late for treatment. Five-year cures were obtained in eight of the 19 operable cases, or 40.5 per cent, while 30 of the 181 inoperable and borderline, or 16.6 per cent, remained symptomatically cured five years later. There were five deaths immediately following treatment, or 1.2 per cent of the total number of 905 cases.

Less glowing accounts of radium cures have been reported in America. Bailey and Healy,[61] in 1923, reported the follow-up study of 908 cases of uterine cancers treated by radium at the Memorial Hospital in New York. In the series there were 11 early operable cervical cancers in which five-year study was permissible. Of these, three, or 27 per cent, were alive and free from evidence of cancer for five years or more. This percentage of cures is probably lower than the actual fact since there were three deaths from intercurrent diseases and one following operation in another clinic during the period of the follow-up. There were 33 cases of borderline cervical cancer, of which eight, or 25 per cent, were alive five years after, and all but one were known to be free from evidence of the disease. There were 123 advanced primary cervical cancers, of which eight, or 6½ per cent, were alive five years later.

Clark and Block,[62] in 1924, reported the results of radium treatment in their series of 144 cervical cancers treated in the University Hospital in Philadelphia. Five-year cures were obtained in 27.2 per cent of 22 operable cases, and in 6.7 per cent of 118 inoperable cases. There were four recurrent inoperable cases with 25 per cent of five-year cures. In the entire series of 144 cases, only 15 per cent of which were operable, there were 10.4 per cent of five-year cures by radium. Clark believes that his results show that while radium has been of the greatest help in the relief of inoperable cases and has effected a cure in a small percentage of those who otherwise are doomed, it nevertheless falls far short of an ideal remedy. The results of his radiation cases compared favorably with those of his radical operations. In such a series of cases treated and reported from his clinic in 1913, there was 33 per cent of five-year cures together with an 8 per cent incidental mortality. In his 22 operable cases treated by radium there was no primary mortality; and only 27.2 per cent five-year cures. Clark says that if the 6.7 per cent of five-year cures of inoperable cases treated by radium is added to the 27.2 per cent of five-year cures by radium in the operable cases the total is practically equivalent to that obtained by radical operation but without the many distressing sequelae incidental to the latter. It appears to us, however, that a better result might have been obtained in the entire series if the early operable cases had been operated and all others had been treated by radium.

Schmitz,[63] in December, 1924, reported his five-year results in a series of 103 cervical carcinoma treated by radium and Roentgen ray. At the end of five years there were living and apparently symptom-free 15 cases, or 14.5 per cent, of the total. Schmitz divided his material into four groups: group one being comprised of the clearly localized single growths for which he believes radical surgical excision is indicated and would have been performed had there not been contraindications for operation; group two containing the operable cases in which there was a suspicion of beginning invasion of the tissue surrounding the growth, and which he believes should be treated with radium and Roentgen ray and subsequent radical surgical excision; group three containing the cases ordinarily considered inoperable, the treatment for which is radium and Roentgen ray; and group four, comprised of the late inoperables with extensive involvement and distant metastases for which palliative and symptomatic treatment alone was recommended. Schmitz states that he has living five years after beginning treatment all three of the three early operable cases of group one, which were treated only by radium and Roentgen ray; six, or 40 per cent, of the 15 later operable cases of group two; six, or 10 per cent, of the 60 inoperable cases of group three; and none of the 25 cases of group four.

In 1924,[64] Greenough presented the preliminary report of a committee appointed by the American College of Surgeons to study the treatment of malignant diseases with radium and Roentgen ray. The material includes 829 cases but will not be considered here because the report is concerned with three-year cures, whereas we feel that, especially with radium cases, it is useless to study anything less than five-year cures.

Our own results may be of some interest, since it is known that the cancer mortality in San Francisco is higher than that of any other city of the United States. During the nine years between July, 1915, and July, 1924, there were 218 carcinoma of the cervix treated in our clinic. Yet we feel that the series is too small to permit of study of five-year cures, a condition shared by nearly all gynecologic clinics, since the results in a small series may be unduly influenced in case they happen to include a few rare cancers which respond unusually well to treatment. Between March, 1916, when we did the first radical operation of the present series, and October, 1923, we had treated 168 uterine cancers by radium or in combination. The series contained 148 carcinoma of the uterine cervix comprising: 114 primary cancers which had not had a previous operation; 34 which had been operated elsewhere and were sent in for prophylactic postoperative radiation or for treatment of recurrence; and 20 carcinoma of the uterine fundus. There were 30 cervical carcinomas which were adjudged primarily operable, a condition which we defined as including not only the very localized growth, but also the early borderline cases in which there were suspicions of parametrial involvement (operability 26 per cent of 114 cases). Operation was refused by two, was contraindicated by systemic conditions in five, and was performed by the Wertheim method in 23, the majority having had either preoperative or postoperative radiation or both. There were four deaths from operation, or 17.33 per cent mortality, including one which died following an operation to close a bladder fistula two months after the primary operation. Another case developed a ureteral fistula. These two cases are the only ones presenting operative trauma which caused difficulty in a series of nearly 50 Wertheim operations. While we do not present our small series from the standpoint of cure, it has helped us to read more intelligently the results of other men who also record their experience with operation and radium. Between March, 1916, and December 30, 1920, we did 19 Wertheim operations with four operative deaths (as an example of the obvious fact that the mortality rate declines with operative experience, it is only fair to state that since that time we have done 15 extensive Wertheim operations with but one death). Four of the remaining 15 cases were subsequently known to have died from cancer, one at nine months, two at one year, and one at three and a half years. There died from intercurrent disease while clinically free from cancer although there was no autopsy, two cases, one from a paralytic stroke in the second year, and one from pneumonia at five years. Four, unfortunately, have escaped from a very vigorous follow-up but were clinically well when last seen, one each at two, two and a half, three, and three and a half years after operation. Five are living and clinically free from cancer, one each at three, four, five, five and a half, and seven years after operation. Therefore, in a series of 19 cases treated by operation, all of which have been followed for between four and eight years there are four cases, or 21 per cent, of the total cases operated which are known to have been clinically well at least five years. This is of interest to us since it is more than likely that there may be finally some other cures in the four cases which have been lost to view and in the two cases which are living and symptom-free short of this five-year period.

We naturally contrast this series with that of our seven operable cases which were treated only by radium and without primary death. One died from a cardiac condition at the end of one year, while symptom-free from cancer; three died from cancer, one each at three, three, and three and a half years after treatment. There were clinically well December, 1924, only three cases, one each at three, four and three-fourths, and five years after treatment. Two only of these seven cases may be considered as cures, although one of them still lacks three months of the five-year period. The result in percentage does not seem to admit of much future improvement since there is only one other of the seven cases which is still living.

Although our results in inoperable cases are not arranged for study of the five-year period, it does not seem as if we were likely to cure any noticeable percentage by radiation, since of the 80 primary cervical cancers which were only radiated, two were lost from the follow-up, 65 were known to be dead, and there were only 13 living, three in the third, two in the fourth, one in the fifth, and seven less than two years. We have been interested in the fact that five died in the third and seven in the fourth year.

There were 34 cancers of the cervix that were operated elsewhere for which we radiated recurrence. Twenty-nine are dead, and only four lived more than two or less than three and a half years. Five cases still live, one each at two and a half, three, three and a half, and five years.

Our results confirm the view that five years' freedom from recurrence is the minimum which can be considered a cure. Thus, in our operative series, only one case lived three and a half years but succumbed to cancer; the three operable cases that were treated only by radium survived between three and three and a half years before succumbing to the disease. Also one so-called recurrence after operation which we treated by radium lived three and a half years. These would have been counted cures in a three-year standard.

*Roentgen Ray Supplemental to Radium in Treatment of Cancer.*—The question is frequently debated as to what extent the deep Roentgen ray contributes to the cures of cases treated primarily with radium. Little help can be obtained from the older literature because of the great improvements that have been made in Roentgen ray during this time. Zweifel,[65] in a meeting of the German Gynecologic Congress, in 1922, stated that the results of Doederlein during the years 1917 and 1919 were improved by the addition of Roentgen ray only from 48 per cent to 54 per cent for operable cases and from 6 per cent to 7 per cent for inoperable cases, but we feel that very much more can be obtained at the present time. The fact that deep Roentgen ray alone occasionally cures is shown by Bumm's report in 1922 that he had cured for five years or more, three, or 13.6 per cent, of 22 operable cancers. The addition of deep Roentgen ray to vaginal extirpations increased the percentage of cures in Amann's [66] clinic in Munich, up to 1923, from 39 per cent to 61 per cent, for a series only one-fifth of which had been observed for five years. While it is undoubtedly true that the literature does not show what can be accomplished by the addition of modern Roentgen ray to radium treatment of cervical cancers, there are few at the present time that do not consider it a necessary adjunct.

*Treatment of Cervical Cancers.*—The literature of the past few years proves that radium cures: a small percentage of absolutely inoperable growths; more borderline cases than surgery; and about the same number of operable cases as surgery is reported to do. It insists that this is

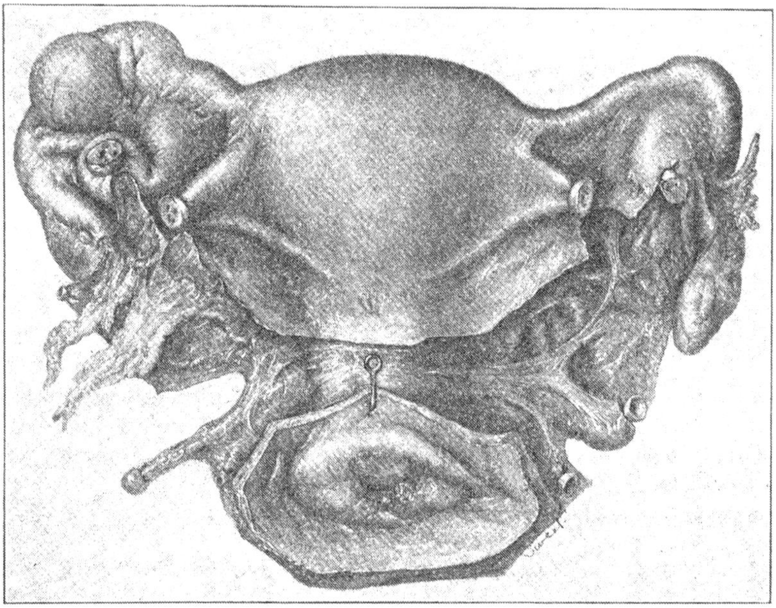

Fig. 2.—Illustrating Extensive Dissection and Removal of Parametrium and Broad Ligament in a Radical Operation for Early Cervical Carcinoma. The uterine vessels have been ligated almost at their point of origin and the ureter has been freed from its bed. There was a double ureter on the right side.

accomplished without noticeable primary mortality, a prolonged hospital stay, or serious postoperative sequelæ. It urges that the technic of radium treatment is constantly improving, and that the results at the present time are by no means as good as may be obtained in a few years, especially if the radium treatment is supplemented with the deep Roentgen ray therapy. For these reasons, the advocates feel that surgery should be abandoned in favor of radium in the treatment of cervical cancers.

There is no doubt but that this contention is true, assuming that the treatment is conducted by one skilled in the use of radium and that the surgical treatment is in the hands of men who are not doing truly radical operations. If the surgeon practices only the ordinary abdominal or vaginal panhysterectomy, we feel that the case will do better with radium followed by Roentgen ray than by such operative procedures.

Personally, however, we are not at all convinced that radium should be used rather than surgery in the treatment of early cervical cancers, provided a truly radical operation is done (Fig. 2). This opinion is based upon our own experience confirmed by study of the literature. We are much interested in the fact that Heymann, while curing 16.6 per cent of 181 inoperable and borderline cases in Stockholm, cured only eight of 19 operable cases in a city in which surgery had been abandoned in favor of radium because of the excellence of the radium results. And in the report of Clark, who cured but five of the 22 operable cases which he radiated, and in our own series in that we are not likely to cure more than two of seven truly operable cases. The fact that radium does not cure 100 per cent of local growths suggests that there is more to the cure of the cancer than the destruction of the tumor by radium, and it is the action on the system by the radium which produces curing factors which are vital to the success of the treatment. No one can believe that inoperable cancers are cured solely by the action of radium upon the tumor cells, since there are often cancer cells far beyond the reach of the rays. It seems logical to believe that a protective substance has developed in the body in reaction to the tumor which aids in marked degree the local effect of radium on the cancer mass, and that nature has not yet developed its protective mechanism in the small early growths. The tumor in two of our operable cases treated by radium was extremely small, and we feel confident that, had surgery been possible, it would have resulted in a cure.

We do not feel that the literature at the present time contains a report of enough operable cases treated by radium to warrant any definite opinion as to whether surgery or radium is the better method. There are only 150 operable cases in the literature we have cited above with 52 per cent of cures. Yet the percentages of cures vary tremendously, from 27 per cent for the series of Clark and of Bailey, to 80 per cent for Doederlein and 100 per cent for Schmitz. Detailed study of the reports show that, with the exception of the Doederlein series, the maximum number of cases in any one series is 22, while another series had only three cases. Thus Seitz reported eight operable cases with four cures; Beuttner, nine operable cases with four cures; Heymann, 19 cases with eight cures; Bailey and Healy, 11 cases with three cures; Clark, 22 cases with five cures; Schmitz, three cases with three cures; Doederlein, 43 operable cases completely radiated with 35 five-year cures, and 34 operable cases incompletely radiated with 15 cures. The latter series was the one whose patients felt so greatly improved that they did not return for the rest of the treatment. Doederlein's complete series of operable cases shows 65 per cent of five-year cures. Were others able to equal this percentage, there would be no doubt of the superiority of the radium. Yet the 72 cases reported by Seitz, Beuttner, Heymann, Bailey and Healy, Clark, and Schmitz gave only 27 cures, or 37½ per cent.

Truly radical surgery has accomplished far more. Von Franqué's[67] report showed 80 per cent surgical cures for five to eight years, Faure[68] cured 50 per cent of 71 cases but more than 80 per cent of the very early cases, while Bumm in a larger series obtained 49 per cent or 77 cases out of 157 operated who were cured for six to eight years, and Wertheim's older series of 160 cases living and well out of 380 who were operated five or more years before, 43 per cent. The small but remarkable series of Ries is cited in the text. These points reënforce us in the opinion we gave in 1919[69] that only the early and truly operable cases should be treated by very radical surgery and that all others should be treated by radium and the deep Roentgen ray (Fig. 3). We feel, however, that all

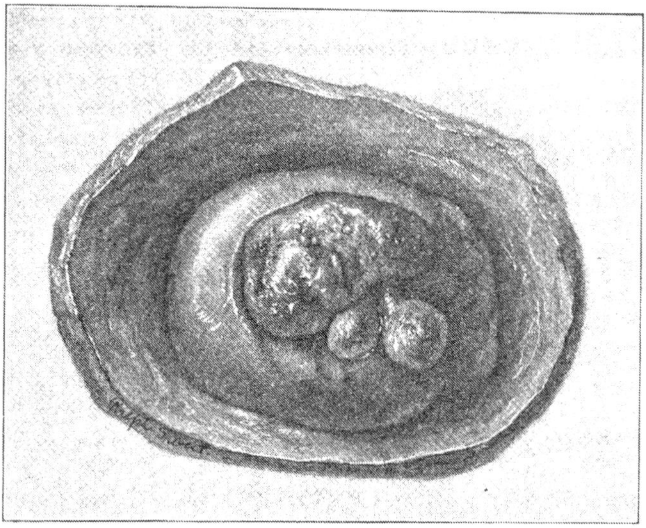

FIG. 3.—ILLUSTRATING WIDE AREA OF VAGINAL RESECTION ESSENTIAL WITH OPERABLE CERVICAL CARCINOMA. (The patient is living and free from subjective and objective findings five years after operation.)

cases should have deep Roentgen ray therapy as a supplementary treatment, no matter whether the case was treated primarily by operation or radium. Moreover, we radiate all cases two weeks before operation with approximately 2000 mc.-hours. At the present time, we are much interested in the technic of Heymann to whose articles[60] we refer those interested.

**Carcinoma of the Uterine Body.**—Norris and Vogt,[70] in 1924, as a result of an exhaustive study of 115 cases confirmed our belief at the time the text went to press that the treatment of choice of carcinoma of the uterus is operation and not radium, the operation being supplemented by postoperative irradiation.

**Ovarian Carcinoma.**—In marked contrast to cervical cancers, the literature is indicating that there may be occasionally a hope of curing by surgical removals some ovarian carcinoma that have been incompletely removed by surgery, if the cases are subsequently treated with the deep Roentgen ray (Fig. 3). This method occasionally gives better results than the Roentgen ray therapy alone, since the rays do not appear to act well until most of the cancer has been removed by surgery. While it is not possible to talk of five-year cures at the present time, we have had several striking results which were at least distinctly palliative. One of our cases, an incomplete removal, lived more than one year, dying from an aplastic anemia. No cancer cells were found at autopsy. The question naturally arises as to whether the Roentgen ray treatment contributed to the anemia, yet the case is most interesting.

**Chorionepithelioma.**—On page 319 of *Pelvic Neoplasms,* we cite a chorionepithelioma reported by Rockafellow in which, after removal of the uterus, metastases developed in the labia. Sometimes they were as large as a kidney and, when excised, returned in a week or so. After four operations for recurrences, the patient's condition became so bad that it did not seem worth while to again attempt removal. To every one's surprise, the growths began to shrink spontaneously, and the patient improved to regain good health. Rockafellow writes us that this patient was again examined in June, 1923, ten years following operation. There was no sign of recurrence and the patient had gained weight from 84 pounds to 146 and seemed in perfect health.

Such cases, although extremely rare, together with the few cases of ovarian cancer which occasionally have improved remarkably after incomplete removal and Roentgen ray treatment, serve to emphasize the view that the cure in malignant neoplasms is at least partially dependent upon the development in the body of reactionary protective substances, which may be even equal to the local treatment.

## LITERATURE

1. Ferguson. Edinb. M. J. Ob. Trans. 1924. 31:149.
2. Fullerton. Surg., Gynec. & Obst. 1925. 243.
3. Attwenger. Arch. f. Gynæk., Berl. 1923. 121:135.
4. Taussig. Am. J. Obst. & Gynec. 1923. 6:407.
5. Lovelace. J. Am. M. Ass. 1923. 80:375.
6. Schellekens. Nederl. Tijdschr. v. Geneesk., Haarlem. 1923. 67, Pt. 2:1212.
7. Taussig. Diseases of the Vulva. D. Appleton & Co. 1923. 223.
8. Bailey and Bagg. Am. J. Obst. 1921. 2:587.
9. Keene. Am. J. Obst. 1921. 2:650.
10. E. Zweifel. Arch. f. Gynæk. 1922. No. 117:269.
11. Schmitz. Surg., Gynec. & Obst. 1924. 39:775.
12. O'Neil. J. Urol. 1921. 5:325.
13. Venot and Parcelier. Rev. de chir. 1921. 59:565.
14. Pomeroy. Surg., Gynec. & Obst. 1922. 35:355.
15. O'Conor. J. Urol. 1924. 159.
16. Shaw. J. Obst. & Gynæc. Brit. Emp. 1923. 30:215.
17. Falls. Am. J. Obst. & Gynec. 1923. 6:673.

18. Pfeiffer. Arch. f. Gynæk. 1923. 120:305.
19. Veit. Ztschr. f. Geburtsh. u. Gynäk. 1924. 87:422.
20. Stacy. Am. J. Roentgenol. 1922. 9:48.
21. Dellepiane. Ann. di ostet. 1924. 46:197.
22. Schleussner. Proc. N. York Path. Soc. 1924. 2133.
23. Sampson. Arch. Surg. 1921. 3:245.
24. Herly. Surg., Gynec. & Obst. 1924. 39:626.
25. Lynch. Calif. State J. M. 1923. November.
26. Lawson. Calif. & Western Med. 1925. March.
27. Werner. München. med. Wchnschr. 1921. June, 24.
28. Stacy. Am. J. Roentgenol. 1922. 9:658.
29. Naujoks. Ztschr. f. Geburtsh. u. Gynäk. 1923. 86:638.
30. Essen-Moeller. Rev. franç. de gynéc. et d'obstet. J. Am. M. Ass., 1922. 78:471.
31. Vogt. Am. J. Obst. & Gynec. 1923. 5:523.
32. Masson. Am. J. Obst. & Gynec. 1923. 5:345.
33. Reed and Charlton. Ann. Surg. 1923. 476.
34. Jeff Miller. Med. & Surg. J. 1924. April.
35. Pennsylvania State Cancer Commission. Campaign Notes of American Society for Control of Cancer. 1924. 6. No. 10.
36. Dartigues. Rev. franç. de Gynec. et d'obstet. 1923. 18:65.
37. Seitz. Deutsche med. Wchnschr. 1922. 48:345.
38. Wintz. Internat. Survey Gyn. 1923. 12:235.
39. Béclère. J. de radiol. et d'électrol. 1921. 5:449.
40. Hanks. J. Radiology. 1924. 5:173.
41. Hempel-Jörgensen. Acta Gynec. Scandin. Helsingfors. 1923. 3:218.
42. Lundquist. Acta Radiol. Stockholm. 1922. 1:524.
43. Warren and Whipple. J. Exper. M. 1923. 38:725-731.
44. Keene. Am. J. Obst. 1924. 8:201.
45. Burnam. Am. J. Obst. 1924. 8:411.
46. Ward. See reference 45.
47. Bailey. See reference 45.
48. Faure. Radiotherapie des fibromes. Bull. mém. Soc. de chir. de Par. 1922. 488:644.
49. Schmid. Ztschr. f. Geburtsh. u. Gynäk. 1923. 86:36.
50. Gouillioud. Gynéc. et obstet., Par. 1924. 9:268.
51. Nuzum. Surg., Gynec. & Obst. 1925. March.
52. Little. Eugenics. 1923. 1:186.
53. Wells. J. Am. M. Ass. 1923. 81:1017.
54. Broders. J. Am. M. Ass. 1920. 74:656.
55. Martzlof. Johns Hopkins Hosp. Bull. 1923. May and June.
56. Pomeroy and Strauss. J. Am. M. Ass. 1924. 83:1060.
57. Von Seuffert. Fortschr. a. d. Geb. d. Röntgenstrahlen. 1922. No. 2. 30:123.
58. Seitz. Wien. klin. Wchnschr. Berlin. 1922. 1:72.
Arch. f. Gynæk. 1923. 117:258.

59. BEUTTNER. Schweiz. med. Wchnschr. 1923. 53:105.
60. HEYMANN. J. Obst. Gynæc. Brit. Emp. 1924. 31:1.
61. BAILEY ANL HEALY. Am. J. Obst. & Gynec. 1923. 6:402.
62. CLARK AND BLOCK. Am. J. Obst. & Gynec. 1924. 7:543.
63. SCHMITZ. Surg., Gynec. & Obst. 1924. December.
64. GREENOUGH. Surg., Gynec. & Obst. 1924. 39:18.
65. ZWEIFEL. See reference 67.
66. AMANN. See reference 67.
67. VON FRANQUÉ. München. med. Wchnschr. 1923. 70:676.
68. FAURE. Abstracted J. Am. M. Ass. 1921. 76:481.
69. LYNCH. Calif. State J. M. 1920. February.
70. NORRIS AND VOGT. Am. J. Obst. & Gynec. 1924. 7:550.

# THE TOXEMIAS OF PREGNANCY

GEORGE WILLIAM KOSMAK, M.D.

## APPENDIX

The general subject of the toxemias of pregnancy continues to occupy professional attention to a large degree. However, since the publication of this volume in 1922, comparatively few noteworthy contributions have been made to medical literature dealing with the etiology and pathology of the several varieties of the toxemias of pregnancy. Certain lines of investigation seem to have been left untouched. Original research in the domain of pathology, for example, has not as yet been extended to the circulatory system or to the endocrines and the hope may be recorded that the next decade will throw some light on etiological factors based on a possible disturbance in the system of ductless glands. Nor has the nervous system been given the attention which it deserves, for no definite pathologic basis for the irritability, which is such a prominent feature, particularly in the toxemias of the later months of pregnancy, has been discovered. The close association between eclampsia and possible kidney lesions still occupies the center of the stage, but I can add very little to my conception of the subject as detailed in a previous chapter. The fact that toxemias of pregnancy in the later months occur without demonstrable kidney lesions, except a possible insufficiency, shows that we are perhaps inclined to such association by clinical rather than pathologic tests. In this connection attention may be drawn to the concept of this disturbance which has been denominated by Kellogg as a "recurrent toxemia of pregnancy." Kellogg believes that in this particular group of cases of toxemia, the kidney insufficiency is the signal symptom in a recurring pregnancy. It is important to recognize this possible distinction between the class of cases which Kellogg calls by the new term and which I have described under the general title of "nephritic toxemia," because in making such distinction the prognosis can be more definitely determined in the individual case. Kellogg believes that if the condition is recognized, much can be done to avoid future trouble by careful attention to diet, thorough rest, with a minimum of exercise, at least ten hours' sleep every night, and absolute freedom from worry and care. All forms of exercise except moderate walking are interdicted and exposure to wet and cold must be avoided. Kellogg believes that with such care patients may be carried through subsequent pregnancies who have aborted or who have had labor induced for increasing signs of toxemia. I am inclined to agree with this view and have personally observed several instances in which pregnancies have been successfully carried through under this régime and in which no definite evidences of kidney pathology could be elicited.

**Treatment.**—In so far as the treatment of the toxemias of pregnancy is concerned no noteworthy results have been accomplished although it may be recorded that the last two years have shown even more conclusively the advantages of conservative treatment, particularly in the convulsive types of the disease. Taking up first, however, the disturbances in the early months, including vomiting, there seems to be a consensus of opinion that the restriction of proteids and fats in the food, with an excess of carbohydrates supplemented by intravenous injections of glucose, have done much to bring about improvement and even cure. The insistence of a carbohydrate diet is enough in many cases to turn the tide, together with the administration of sufficient alkalies and sedatives where the latter are needed. Speaking in greater detail, I am accustomed to prescribe carefully just what articles of diet are suitable and include here the free use of cereals of all kinds, breadstuffs, and milk in moderate quantities, without cream. In addition, green vegetables of all kinds, including the free use of lettuce, celery, radishes, and fresh fruits. As the latter may cause indigestion they are best taken well cooked, with sugar to flavor. Bowel evacuations are essential and should be secured with simple cathartics. As these patients are more or less dehydrated from the constant vomiting, the use of salines is contraindicated and the simpler vegetable cathartics such as cascara in pill form seem to give the best results. Alkalies are well borne at this time, and there are now on the market a number of pleasant and palatable preparations which can be administered without distress to the patient. The use of milk sugar I have found of great service as it is less sweet than the cane variety and borne in larger quantities. I give it in a weak lemonade in the proportion of a well-rounded tablespoonful to the pint of water flavored with the juice of half a lemon. At least three pints of this agreeable drink can be taken during the course of twenty-four hours and the water seems much more easily retained in this form than when taken plain. I have already alluded in a previous chapter to the intravenous administration of sugar solution in the advanced cases of hyperemesis and my experience during the past two years confirms the good results previously obtained. A 5 or 10 per cent carefully sterilized solution of glucose administered in quantities of from 500 to 1000 c.c., frequently turns the tide in the patient's favor. The danger of glycosuria has often been referred to in cases of high carbohydrate feeding or sugar instillation, and while I have occasionally observed traces of sugar in the urine after the latter, these are transitory. Of course in the presence of a true diabetes the question of sugar instillation or exclusive carbohydrate feeding must be carefully considered and in the presence of a true diabetes as confirmed by a high blood sugar content, the question of abortion must be immediately considered if the use of insulin does not immediately provoke a good result.

Further studies in the combined use of insulin and glucose for the treatment of excessive vomiting of pregnancy have recently been contributed by Thalhimer, who now reports eight cases successfully treated by this means. In view of the lack of understanding and the limitations of this method of treatment and the indiscriminate use of insulin injections that have come to my personal notice, I desire to call particular attention to the technic of administration. Of course the essential idea is to combat the acidosis resulting from carbohydrate deficiency as near as we now understand this subject. The relationship of insulin to the pancreas is still obscure and the exact mechanism of its action unknown. We do know, however, that it controls diabetes and causes the disappearance of acidosis even in non-diabetic patients. It does this more rapidly, however, when glucose is administered in conjunction with it. In severe cases of hyperemesis the persistent acidosis is the alarming feature and as a vicious cycle has been established by constant vomiting, no relief can be obtained from nutriment administered through the usual channels. The intravenous administration of glucose has, however, apparently solved the problem.

In instituting this line of treatment only sick cases should be considered which have resisted the more conservative measures referred to elsewhere. Such patients should be kept in hospitals and watched closely. It is always advisable, where this can be done, to determine the carbon dioxid combining power of the blood plasma. One hundred c.c. of the chemically pure glucose of some reliable manufacture should be made into a solution with 1000 c.c. of sterile water. The solution should remain colorless after its sterilization in an autoclave. Where a patient is severely dehydrated 200° c.c. of a 5 per cent solution can be given. The essential point is to give it slowly, taking up at least four hours for the administration through a vein in the arm. It is recommended that one unit of insulin be given for approximately every 3 grams of glucose. Thus for 100 grams, 30 units of insulin are given in divided doses; 20 one hour after beginning the glucose infusion and 10 units after the second hour. In the cases thus far studied it has been found that the ketonuria is relieved in from six to eight hours. The treatment can be repeated at intervals of from one to two days depending on the patient's response and as soon as vomiting stops the administration of food by mouth should be begun.

**Uric Acid.**—In a study of the uric acid content of amniotic fluid, Williams and Bargen found this as well as creatinin present in appreciable amounts. Although the concentration does not appear to vary in relation to any particular pathologic condition, the highest values were found in the fluid from a case of toxic vomiting. The uric acid was also found to increase with the termination of pregnancy and the highest point (7.73 Mgms. per 100 c.c.) was found in a case three weeks overdue, which leads to the supposition that the fetal urine may be a source of the same. Williams and Bargen conclude that the greater concentration of uric acid in the amniotic fluid over that in the blood suggests that in the toxemia of pregnancy the increased uric acid in the blood may arise in part from a more highly saturated amniotic fluid. If this is true, the rapid subsidence of toxic symptoms after rupture of the membranes in many cases may be partially accounted for.

Further studies in the uric acid content of the blood have also been presented by King and Denis, who compared their observation in normal and toxic cases and found that, while their results confirmed those of Williams, Caldwell, and Killian, they were not able to differentiate between renal and hepatic toxemias as claimed by the latter. However, in preëclamptic states, King and Denis believe that the increased blood uric acid may serve as a useful test in doubtful cases, for the more toxic patients showed high uric acid values associated with a relatively small rise in the nonprotein nitrogen.

Edema.—Since Zangemeister presented in 1919 his theory that the retention of water in the tissues is a causative factor in the production of eclampsia, comparatively little attention has been paid to this idea. He claimed that the primary cause of the edema is an injury to the capillary endothelium, which manifests itself in increased permeability and diminished absorptive ability, although he maintains that these changes are only indirectly associated with the etiology of eclampsia. The infiltration of the tissues is accompanied by a rise in blood pressure and elimination of albumin through the kidneys, while the edema of the brain results in convulsions and coma. Others have confirmed the occurrence of this definite blood dilution even in normal pregnancy but in the late toxemias this is even more marked and proportional to the extent of the edema; in other words, the more evident the swelling the lower the protein concentration in the blood. The clinical observation has likewise been made that patients with extreme edema present a better prognosis, so that it may be argued that the general retention of water is a prophylactic measure adopted by the organism. Plass, who has written an excellent review of the metabolic disturbances occurring during the eclamptic state, points out that this plasma dilution may explain certain other findings which are otherwise difficult to interpret. For example, the very low values for the non-protein nitrogen constituents generally found in normal pregnancy and frequently in the toxemias may thus be regarded as the result of a simple dilution, while the increased percentage of chlorides may be looked upon as a mechanism for maintaining the osmotic pressure of the blood, which would otherwise be abnormally low.

**Toxicity.**—An interesting contribution to the pathogenesis of eclampsia has been made by Levi-Solal and Tzanck. By animal experimentation these investigators have found that serum from eclamptic women is toxic to guinea pigs in the proportion of 1 to 2 c.c. per kilo of body weight, while such animals are not affected by male serum or that from normal women even if pregnant, or from other animals notwithstanding doses six or eight times as large. This observation is in confirmation of what has already been reported by Barr and others. Moreover they believe that eclamptic serum contains two toxic principles, one of which is capable of producing convulsions, and the other, while equally lethal is not convulsant. The former seems to be rendered innocuous by heating to 55° C. or by disintoxicating the eclamptic by treatment. The other principle, however, is not thus dissipated and is found in the serum of former eclamptics or of albuminuric women with hypertension, and in other conditions.

In other words, these facts seem to show that a part of the eclamptic toxemia is due to organic alterations which result in the production of the two toxic substances. Animals which have been subjected to the injection of these materials develop a typical eclampsia with convulsions which is rapidly fatal where the first toxic principle is employed, whereas the administration of the second makes the animals torpid and they finally die without having had convulsions. These authors are therefore of the opinion that the phenomena of eclampsia are identical with those of anaphylactic shock, because of the suddenness of the onset, the possible recurrence in successive gestations, and the frequent disappearance of symptoms with intrauterine fetal death. Efforts to trace the origin of these toxins to placental villi were successful in so far as unautolysed filtrates from the placentae of eclamptics produced effects identical with those following the administration of eclamptic serum. The authors believe that drugs acting on the sympathetic nervous system would afford a protection against eclampsia, for pilocarpine hydrochlorid in the dose of 1 Mg. for a guinea pig of 500 Gms., when mixed with a lethal dose of eclamptic serum or of placental extract prevented the death of the animal in over 80 per cent of the cases. Adrenalin, atropin, and eserin were likewise employed but no protective effect elicited. The clinical application of this method was possible in only one case, a patient who had had nine convulsions before the injection of 5 Mgms. of pilocarpin, which was repeated three times in the first twenty-four hours although no further convulsions had occurred after the first dose.

**Incidence of Eclampsia.**—An interesting commentary on the incidence of eclampsia is presented in a report to the British Congress of Obstetricians and Gynecologists, in June, 1922, which is commented upon by Eden. It seems that there are about 600 deaths from eclampsia annually in Great Britain and Ireland and from an average mortality of about 22 per cent Eden estimates the incidence to be, therefore, about 3000 cases per annum. The maternal mortality rate varied from about 11 to 25 per cent and although the disease is less common in multiparae, the maternal mortality is higher. It seems that the high fetal mortality is due more to prematurity than to the toxemia of the mother, likewise the narcotics; the usually forcible delivery and the deprivation of breast milk are additional factors. Commenting on the method of treating, Eden points out that natural delivery assisted or induced, yields results twice as favorable as those following cesarean section. Accouchement forcé in all cases carried a mortality from two to five times higher than similar cases handled by more conservative measures, from which he concludes that in all cases whether mild or severe, a minimum of obstetric interference is indicated and that the methods advocated by Stroganoff and Tweedy are among the most available and satisfactory to date.

**Etiology.**—Chronic sepsis as the etiological factor in the production of the toxemias of pregnancy has previously been alluded to (page 34) and J. E. Talbot has presented another paper more recently, in which he claims to show that the placental infarct is the result of hematogenous infection of the placental site, dating primarily from a point of absorption in the teeth or tonsils. His reasoning to substantiate these claims is rather lengthy but he believes that the usual symptoms of eclampsia, either with or without convulsions, are those which may be attributed to the manifestations of a septic process and that the fundamental principles upon which this conception is based are equally applicable to other infectious complexes.

**Lazard Treatment.**—The intravenous use of magnesium sulphate in puerperal eclampsia constitutes the subject of a preliminary report by Lazard (*Am. J. Obst. & Gynec.*, February, 1925). The sedative action of magnesium sulphate on the nerve cells has been known since the work of Meltzer and Auer in 1904, who employed the drug for the control of tetanic convulsions. Lazard uses 20 c.c. of a 10 per cent solution of magnesium sulphate by intravenous injection as soon after the first convulsion as possible, in addition to the usual eliminatory methods, employed, however, with the least possible handling of the patient. Lazard reports a series of 17 cases with but one maternal death, all of which were profoundly toxic, having convulsions and in coma when first seen. Among these were 11 antepartum cases, one in labor, and five postpartum. All of them had one or more convulsions and even where the other measures were not employed, the good results following the magnesium sulphate injections were apparent. The convulsions seemed to be controlled by the sedative effect on the voluntary muscles and no deleterious effect was noted in so far as respiratory or other paralyses were concerned. It was also found that magnesium sulphate in addition to controlling the convulsions undoubtedly reduced the edema by promoting diuresis and thus eliminating toxins. Except for some urgent obstetric indication in eclampsia, surgical interference should not be undertaken. The author is also disposed to recommend the intravenous use of magnesium sulphate in cases of so-called preëclamptic toxemia, which do not improve under the usual treatment, in the hope that the toxemia can be controlled and the pregnancy carried to spontaneous labor without the supervention of an eclamptic seizure. He has not observed any effect on labor itself, either hastening its onset or interfering with its progress after it starts.

**Stroganoff Treatment.**—The Stroganoff method of treating eclampsia and its modifications has continued to gain in favor during recent years and Stroganoff attempted a practical demonstration in London about a year ago. He presented before the British Association of Obstetricians and Gynecologists his most recent summary for which he collected over 2000 cases from various European clinics with a maternal mortality of 9.8 per cent. He claims that the method yields an average infant mortality of only 18 per cent and insists that the details of its execution will materially improve the results already obtained.

Stroganoff's method has been carefully investigated by H. J. Stander of Johns Hopkins University. Stander's observations of Stroganoff's material seemed to show that his results represent the lowest mortality of any large series of cases but is of the opinion that most of the cases personally treated by Stroganoff were relatively mild as compared with those observed in other clinics, because an exceptionally large proportion had no convulsions, or only one, and only a relatively small proportion had more than five convulsions. More or less confusion still exists, however, in various clinics as to the true interpretation of Stroganoff's methods and although the German clinics seem to follow his directions more closely, still there is much divergence. This likewise applies to France. In order to fix firmly in the minds of my readers the Stroganoff treatment as insisted upon by the author, the details of his method are presented herewith. (1) Upon admission: (*a*) Dark room with minimum of noise. (*b*) Special nurse. (*c*) Examination or disturbance of patient only when absolutely necessary, and then usually under chloroform. (*d*) 0.015 (0.01-0.02) Gm. morphin hypodermically, while under chloroform narcosis, usually about 10 to 15 Gms. of chloroform being employed. (2) One hour after admission: 2.0 (1.5-2.5) Gms. chloral hydrate per rectum with 100 c.c. normal salt solution and 100 c.c. milk. Should the patient be conscious the chloral hydrate can be administered by mouth with 100 c.c. milk.[1] (3) Three

[1] Chloral hydrate is always administered without the use of chloroform, except where the patient has had one or more convulsions after admission; then about 10 Gms. of the anesthetic are used with each dose of chloral hydrate.

hours after admission: 0.015 (0.01-0.02) Gm. morphin hypodermically under 10 to 15 Gms. chloroform. (4) Seven hours after admission: 2.0 (1.5-2.5) Gms. chloral hydrate, as above. (5) Thirteen hours after admission: 1.5 (1.0-2.0) Gms. chloral hydrate, as above. (6) Twenty-one hours after admission: 1.5 (1.0-2.0) grams chloral hydrate, as above. (7) After each convulsion oxygen is administered as quickly as possible. This is kept up until the breathing improves, usually for about five minutes. (8) after three convulsions in the clinic: venesection of not more than 400 c.c. is resorted to. (9) In case of frequent convulsions chloroform and chloral hydrate to be used more energetically than outlined above. (10) If patient has been free from fits for twenty-four hours or longer after admission, and has not yet been delivered, she should be given about 0.5 Gms. chloral hydrate every eight hours for about three days. (11) Operative delivery is resorted to only when intervention becomes absolutely necessary for the sake of the child.

This method, as outlined, is followed in all cases of eclampsia during labor. In antepartum eclampsia, the same procedure is used except that usually it is advisable to employ smaller quantities of the narcotics. Stroganoff believes that postpartum eclampsia is easier to treat and accordingly recommends the same treatment as in the mild type.

**Williams-Stander Treatment.**—A modification of the Stroganoff procedure is now being tried out in the service of Professor J. W. Williams at Johns Hopkins. Stander, his associate, claims, and in this I am inclined to agree with him, that a moderate rise of blood-pressure should facilitate osmosis and elimination, and represents, therefore, a protective mechanism. Venesection of small quantities of blood such as are advocated by Stroganoff can have little material value in lowering blood-pressure or eliminating toxins and if this method is employed at all at least from 700 to 1000 c.c. of blood should be abstracted. It is of interest to present the details of the methods of treatment now employed at Johns Hopkins Hospital in eclamptic patients:

*Outpatient.*—Patients with increasing blood-pressure and definite trace of albumin must visit the dispensary twice a week. If they do not follow directions, the Social Service must visit them promptly.

*Dispensary.*—Patients must be sent into the hospital whenever they show: (*a*) systolic pressure of 150 or more and + + albumin; (*b*) undue rise in diastolic pressure; (*c*) any one of the foregoing symptoms associated with severe headache, epigastric pain, or pronounced edema; (*d*) sudden amaurosis (loss of vision), even if none of the conditions mentioned previously are present.

*Ward Service.*—TOXEMIAS.—(1) In moderately sick patients when the albumin does not fall to below one gram per liter within a week, or when the general condition is not satisfactory, the induction of labor should be seriously considered. (2) Very ill patients will probably have induction of labor sooner, immediate induction when amaurosis develops suddenly, either with or without epigastric pain. In nulliparae with a rigid cervix, cesarean section may be considered. ECLAMPSIA.—(1) Upon admission: Patients with frank eclampsia are: (*a*) to be placed in a quiet, darkened room and to be disturbed as little as possible; (*b*) to have special nurse continuously until definitely out of coma; (*c*) to have ¼ Gm. morphin hypodermically immediately; (*d*) to be catheterized, examined medically and obstetrically, and bled for 200 ccm. under nitrous oxid anesthesia if conscious. The venesection is done only when it is necessary to obtain a blood specimen for research work; (*e*) to be placed on one side, with foot of bed elevated so long as coma persists. Mucus to be swabbed from pharynx as it collects; (*f*) to have water freely when conscious. If patient cannot drink on account of coma or lack of desire, the intravenous administration of 500 c.c. of 5 per cent glucose should be considered; (*g*) not to be delivered until after cervix is fully dilated. Then by the simplest operative means, unless spontaneous delivery seems imminent; (*h*) no chloroform to be used, (*i*) notify the chemical assistants as soon as patient is admitted so that the necessary observations can be made. (2) One hour after admission: If comatose, give 2 Gms. chloral hydrate in 100 c.c. of normal salt solution, and the same quantity of milk per rectum. If conscious the chloral can be administered by mouth in 100 c.c. of milk. (3) Three hours after admission: ¼ gr. morphia hypodermically. (4) Seven hours after admission: 2 Gms. chloral hydrate as above. (5) Thirteen hours after admission: 1.5 Gms. chloral hydrate as above. (6) Twenty-one hours after admission: 1.5 Gms. chloral hydrate as above. General directions: (*a*) While eclamptic patients are under treatment, the assistants and nurses must insist upon the greatest possible quiet; (*b*) catharsis, sweating, or venesection in excess of 200 c.c. must not be employed.

## LITERATURE

EDEN. J. Obst. & Gynæc. Brit. Emp., 29, 368.
KING, E. L., AND DENIS, W. Am. J. Obst. & Gynec., 1924, 7, 409.
LAZARD, E. M. Am. J. Obst. & Gynec., 1925, 9, 178.
LEVI-SOLAL AND TZANCK, A. Presse méd., 1923, 669, Aug. 1.
PLASS, E. D. Am. J. Obst. & Gynec., 1923, 6, 637.
SELLHEIM, H. Med. Klin., 1923, 9, 1143.
STANDER, H. J. Am. J. Obst. & Gynec., 1925, 9, 327.
TALBOT, J. E. Am. J. Obst. & Gynec., 1923, 6, 709.
THALHIMER, WILLIAM. J. Am. M. Ass., 1924, 82, 696.
——— Surg., Gynec. & Obst., 1924, 39, 237.
WILLIAMS, J. L., AND BARGEN, J. A. Am. J. Obst. & Gynec., 1924, 7, 406.

# STERILITY AND CONCEPTION

CHARLES GARDNER CHILD, JR., M.D.

## APPENDIX

Since this book was written, a wealth of clinical facts and fancies has been published on the subject of sterility. Much of this is of interest, some of great value, and the field is being constantly enlarged by almost daily contributions.

On this hitherto little understood subject much new light has been cast, so that those who to-day are still inclined to discredit the treatment of sterility would do well to stop and explore the evidence so fast accumulating. *Fertility and Sterility in Human Marriages,* by Reynolds, Macomber, and Young is the one book of outstanding importance.

**Rubin Test.**—In the literature of the past two years, one finds much attention paid to the Rubin test, with numerous modifications of his technic, and several new methods not without merit. The substitution of carbon dioxid gas for oxygen, it being more rapidly absorbed, has met with marked favor. Several investigators have reported the use of fluids to ascertain the patency of the tubes. Stone forces either an iodine, or mercuric bichloride solution through the uterus and tubes, using a large glass syringe. His test is performed on the operating table at the time the abdomen is open, with the tube held outside the peritoneal cavity, and he reports no unfavorable results. It would seem highly improbable that gas will be supplanted by fluids for use in testing the patency of tubes, but it may prove of value in certain selected cases.

In placing at their true valuation the conclusions drawn from a Rubin test, it should not be lost sight of that they can never be absolute, and that all other findings must be given their due consideration. With these facts constantly in mind, the transuterine insufflation of gas to determine the patency or stenosis of the fallopian tubes becomes a valuable adjunct in the investigation of sterility in the female. It has been performed with almost complete freedom from harmful effects in thousands of cases in the various gynecological clinics in this country and abroad, and has yielded information unobtainable in any other way. The method is to-day essentially as when first introduced in 1919, despite numerous suggestions for modification and simplification that have been made by different workers. (For description of both apparatus and technic see monograph by Rubin in this series.)

*Interpretation.*—Pressure findings, fluoroscopic examination, and shoulder pain give the data from which conclusions are drawn. The first is the most important, and from it one may conclude that both tubes are freely open when gas passes into the abdomen at a pressure of 100 or less. If more than 100, but less than 150, no definite conclusions can be drawn regarding the condition of the tubes, and further investigation by other methods must be used. Only 13 per cent of 600 cases tested by Aldridge fell into this class, which he regards as the indefinite group. A pressure above 150 points unquestionably to definite obstruction in one or both tubes, and when the mercury rises to 200 without a drop, the test may be concluded and the tubes regarded as in a state of total occlusion. In normal cases in the upright position the gas can be seen as a clear layer beneath the diaphragm when the case is examined fluoroscopically. However, a low pressure combined with shoulder pains is proof enough of the presence of gas in the abdomen, and the only advantage of the fluoroscope is in those cases where a drop in pressure is not followed by pain. Pain is almost uniformly present in normal cases, and is probably due to the irritation of the phrenic nerve ending in the upper peritoneum where the gas settles; if carbon dioxid is used it disappears upon absorption of gas in about an hour's time.

The test should *not* be performed upon patients with acute or subacute pelvic inflammation, or upon those with advanced cardiac disease, and should be timed as regards the menstrual cycle so that the endometrium will be in the quiescent stage; otherwise a thickened and congested endometrium might give rise to partial tubal stenosis and a resultant false impression. From four days to a week after the last day of the menstrual period, the period that Rubin terms the "post-menstrual phase" is best.

The Rubin test has been performed also during the course of laparotomy to determine more accurately the distorted or occluded part of the genital tract. Peterson found by this method that pressures approaching 300 mm. of Hg were frequently accompanied by rupture of the tube which occurred in the infundibular portion.

Substances opaque to the x-ray, such as sodium bromid solution, have been used in the place of gas as the insufflating medium to facilitate the radiographic study and give more exact information as to the anatomy in the individual case. So far the information yielded by this method has not proved to be of much practical value.

As a therapeutic measure in the treatment of sterility, tubal insufflation is questionable. Peterson reports a number of patients subjected to insufflation of the tubes for diagnostic purposes that subsequently became pregnant, though not for some time after the test. It would seem quite probable that in late conception after tubal insufflation in cases of sterility the delay is due to the establishment of only a very small opening at the time of the test.

*Modifications.*—The modifications of Rubin's method and new methods reported are many, and some have considerable value. Heaney uses a plain, one ounce, all rubber ear syringe. If after the syringe is half empty the air refuses to pass he concludes that the tubes are closed. Ferguson adds a right-angle glass tube, to the offset of which is attached a tube running to the manometer and the bulb near the tip to prevent the escape of air from the uterus. Dickinson uses a glass cannula or standard Rubin intrauterine tube connected by a T with any standard portable manometer and a bulb of 20 c.c. capacity. Bonney has devised a Fenton dilator, size No. 7, with a channel running from end to end and closed during introduction by a stylet. Attached by means of an air-tight push joint is a rubber tube and bulb which connects by a T-piece with the manometer like that used with the sphygmomanometer. He makes the test under anesthesia, using the perforated No. 7 Fenton as a cervical dilator. Several authors make mention of insufflation by means of a Luer syringe used at the fimbriated end of the tube at the time of operation.

Radiography as an adjunct to tubal insufflation would not seem to be necessary unless possibly in an endeavor to determine the location of the obstruction. A most interesting and valuable paper on the subject is contributed by Kennedy who after filling the uterus and tubes with a 20 per cent solution of bromid of sodium, accomplished by means of a compression apparatus, takes the roentgenogram. If the ampulla of the tube does not appear, then either the tube has been removed or there is an obstruction in the isthmus or cornu. He found about twice the number of closures at the fimbria as at the isthmus (69.2 per cent to 30.8 per cent), and deems his method of value in determining before operation the length, breadth, and direction of any tube casting a shadow; the site of any occlusion, or the presence of contained fluid. When no contraindication exists, such as active cervical or tubal involvement, he believes that carbon dioxid insufflation should begin the tubal study.

**Causes of Sterility.**—Many papers have appeared on the *causes* of sterility in the female, but have brought out little new or of much value, and the same may be said about those on *diagnosis*.

Frank has described the florid, hirsute, male type of woman, with large clitoris, congested vulva and cervix, neuter pelvic conformation, large, soft uterus and short uterosacral ligaments, as proverbially unfertile. The same, he says, holds true of pale, flabby, infantile women with rudimentary breasts, small vulva or narrow, short, anteflexed uterus with long conical cervix and narrow fornices.

The most important test for sterility in the male or female, writes Huhner, is the one devised by himself, and which he describes as follows: The examination is to be made as soon as possible after coitus. With a bivalve speculum the cervix is brought into view and some of the cervical contents sucked up in a pipet, immediately expelled on a slide and examined under the microscope. The presence of numerous, lively spermatozoa is definite positive evidence. If only dead spermatozoa are found a condom specimen is examined, and if with the same result, the fault is fixed on the husband. The finding of live spermatozoa in the condom specimen indicates that something about the genital secretion of the female has destroyed them in direct coitus.

Dabney does not believe that the finding of a few viable spermatozoa absolves the man from responsibility, and that a complete physical examination of both partners should initiate every study of sterility in a given mating, since he feels that the general health is often a very real factor. While the rôle of the unbalanced diet has yet to be proven in human reproductivity, though clearly demonstrated in rats, it should nevertheless receive consideration. The reproductive systems and secretions of both parties should be examined in detail. Dabney further lays down as absolute and demonstrable requirements for conception in every woman the possession of essential sex organs, fully developed. One tube must be patent, and miscroscopic examination of the cervical fluid after coitus should show motile spermatozoa.

Several writers discuss the relation between obesity and sterility, and their observations would seem to indicate that the sterility in these cases is probably caused by hypofunction of the ovaries, the obesity occurring secondarily as the result of the ovarian hypofunction.

That exogenous adiposity has little or nothing to do with sterility, while endogenous, primary pituitary or thyroid adiposity may, in view of the reciprocal interactivity of the various endocrine glands, ultimately result in some destructive involvement of the ovaries, leading to sterility, is the opinion advanced by Dietrich, who believes the thyroid and pituitary extracts of some therapeutic value.

Pottenger in a paper on the relation existing between the endocrines and sterility considers the genital function stimulated by the ovarian, pituitary, thyroid, and suprarenal secretions, and diminished by the thymus, and at times by the thyroid. Ovarian hyperplasia and hypoactivity leading to sterility are generally caused by the hypoactivity of the thyroid or pituitary, and sometimes the adrenals. Thyroid deficiency in the early years, he believes, retards the development of the sex organs, and in later life, depresses the functions of ovulation and menstruation, tending to sterility. These cases are to be helped by the administration of thyroid substance. Pottenger further states that hypopituitarism before puberty may produce infantilism, both general and sexual, without any marked adiposity, gigantism with adiposity, and genital hypoplasia. All of these, he thinks, lead to sterility because of the hypoplasia, and he recommends the thyroid preparations as giving the best results therapeutically.

Other writers, notably Rongy, express themselves as convinced that organotherapy has no place in the treatment of sterility.

Numerous papers have appeared on the operative and non-operative treatment of sterility. Displacements of the uterus and occlusion of the tubes receive the most attention. Nürnberger uses curettage to permit of the development of a functionally active mucous membrane, and believes it exerts a distinct action on the ovaries. Displacements of the uterus should be corrected, but next to infantilism, tubal obstruction is the most frequent cause of sterility. Groff states that 50 per cent of his cases of sterility showed impermeable tubes, and of these 10 per cent were confirmed by operation. He believes, however, that anomalies of position of the uterus should take first place among operative indications in sterility. Discission and dilatation of the cervix he disapproves of as having little effect on sterility and tending to produce cervical catarrh, and with this Rongy and others agree.

Babcock advocates transplanting the cervix well back in the vaginal fornix and lengthening the anterior vaginal wall when the cervix is long, conical, anteflexed, and accompanied by a short anterior vaginal wall (see page 179 of original volume). He reports a successful case treated in this way. Lynch believes that congenital anomalies account for both sterility and displacement in a very considerable percentage of cases, but that in many of the acquired displacements the disturbance in uterine circulation may be the cause. Many symptomless retro-displacements are of the congenital type, and in these we find sterility more often than in the acquired type.

Aldridge has found in cases of primary sterility that 66.5 per cent showed either partial or complete obstruction of the tubes, and secondary cases 17.4 per cent. In his observation of cases subjected to salpingostomy, subsequent gas insufflation to maintain patency has not been encouraging. From a clinical study of sterility, at Hinkel's, in Vienna, Zimmermann believes that the predominant rôle is played by diseases of the adnexa, and that any cause producing these may ultimately produce sterility. The inhibition of development is only a secondary cause, and general diseases, hormonal disturbances, and inability to produce mature ova are of primary importance, while stenosis of the cervix has only a subordinate bearing, and all treatment should be directed against the original disease, or its results.

Spalding discusses the incidence of venereal diseases in sterility. He found that 16 per cent of the sterility cases gave a positive Wassermann reaction, while the pregnant cases showed only 3.7 per cent. In cases of primary sterility the test is positive in 17 per cent, and in secondary sterility in 14 per cent. These figures agree with the current estimates of syphilitic incidence in sterility.

In the treatment of sterility, artificial insemination receives scant attention. Frank and Nürmberger mention the method only to condemn it, while Meaker reporting a successful case goes more into detail. He believes that the semen should be introduced directly into the cervical canal, and that the specimen used should be perfect as regards number, motility, and morphology of the spermatozoa. The female genital tract above the os externum must likewise be normal. If the mechanical is the only object to be overcome, artificial insemination, he concludes, is satisfactory. Whenever the cervical conditions are hostile to the spermatozoa, it is necessary to inseminate directly into the uterine cavity. Only two drops of semen should be used, and the time of choice he gives as straightway after menstruation has ceased.

Several very excellent contributions on the *prevention* of sterility have appeared. One by Macomber is of especial value. Of great importance is the report of the Committee on Maternal Health of New

York, which makes a strong plea for further inquiry into the subject of contraceptives. Opinions obtained by questionnaire give a very wide difference of opinion among gynecologists and between them and the various birth control clinics, especially those in London and New York. In America, the sheath is the method most used, and for this as high as 12 per cent of failures are reported. Douches alone are discredited, while the chemical suppositories show a lower rate of protection than the jellies, pastes, effervescing tablets of chinosol and acids. The soft rubber cap of Mensinger, fitted over the cervix, by a physician, for the occasion only would seem to give the most protection. The Committee is making further studies along clinical, chemical, and laboratory lines, which should prove of great value in the future.

## LITERATURE

ALDRIDGE. Am. J. Obst. & Gynec. July, 1923.
——— Am. J. Obst. & Gynec. Nov., 1924.
BABCOCK. Am. J. Obst. & Gynec. April, 1923.
BOMPIANI. Ann. di ostet. Milano. Sept., 1924.
BONNEY. Lancet. London, Nov. 22, 1924.
BABNEY. South. M. J. Dec., 1922.
DICKINSON. Am. J. Obst. & Gynec. Nov., 1923.
——— Report of the Committee on Maternal Health of New York.
DIETRICH. Monatschr. f. Geburtsh. u. Gynaek. Berl. Jan., 1923.
FRANK. Proc. Kansas M. Soc. May, 1924.
GRAFF. Arch. f. Gynæk. Berlin. Dec. 20, 1922.
GRAFF AND PETZOLD. Ztschr. f. Geburtsh. u. Gynäk. Stutt. Dec., 1923.
HEANEY. Am. J. Obst. & Gynec. Nov., 1923.
HUHNER. Am. J. Obst. & Gynec. July, 1924.
JACOBY. Surg., Gynec., & Obst. April, 1923.
KENNEDY. Am. J. Obst. & Gynec. July, 1923.
LYNCH. Calif. State J. M. Nov., 1923.
MACOMBER. J. Am. M. Ass. April 7, 1923.
——— Ibid. Aug., 1924.
MEAKER. Boston M. &. S. J. Feb., 1924.
——— Ibid. Sept., 1924.
NURNBERGER. Deutsche med. Wchnschr. Leipz. March 30, April 6, 1923.

PETERSON. Canad. M. Ass. J., Montreal. Dec. 1922. J. Am. M. Ass. Sept., 1923.

POTTENGER. Calif. State J. M. Nov., 1923.

REYNOLDS, MACOMBER. Fertility and Sterility in Human Marriages. Saunders & Co.

RONGY. Am. J. Obst. & Gynec. June, 1923.

SPALDING. Calif. State J. M. Nov., 1923.

STONE. Am. J. Obst. & Gynec. April, 1923.

ZIMMERMANN. Deutsche med. Wchnschr. Leipz. Sept., 1923.

# NON-OPERATIVE TREATMENT IN GYNECOLOGY

GEORGE GELLHORN, M.D.

## APPENDIX

In the short time which has elapsed since this monograph first appeared, no important changes or additions have occurred which would render an extensive revision of the text necessary. A surprisingly large number of letters from almost all parts of the country has demonstrated to me the vivid interest of physicians in the subject presented and the satisfactory results obtained with many of the procedures recommended by me. Particularly numerous have been the inquiries regarding the powder treatment of leukorrhea which clearly indicates that the traditional therapy with douches and curet has proved unsuccessful.

For this reason a brief résumé of the proper treatment of leukorrhea appears desirable.

**Leukorrhea.**—Leukorrhea or, as it is commonly called, vaginal discharge, originates in the vagina itself in only an insignificant number of cases. In the great majority of instances it derives its origin from the cervical canal; less often does it come from the uterine cavity.

The vaginal discharge proper is thin and foamy, and yellow in color if caused by the trichomonas vaginalis, or somewhat thicker in consistence and slightly offensive in odor if saprophytic or other bacteria have been the cause; neglected pessaries or other foreign bodies introduced for contraceptive or masturbation purposes may give rise to a purulent and foul secretion.

The cervical discharge is always thick, grayish in color if purely mucous, but more often with a yellowish tint due to the action of pus-forming microbes; in the earlier stages of gonorrhea it takes on a greenish hue.

The endometrial discharge, finally, is a thin, grayish, yellowish, or colorless fluid. It may represent a hypersecretion of the uterine mucosa due either to endocrine disturbances or to chronic, non-infectious congestions (fibroids, retrodisplacements, subinvolution, etc.), or it may be the end result of a uterine infection of long standing.

With such a variety of causes, sites of origin, and physical properties it is obviously illogical to expect results in every case from one and the same remedy. To institute one's treatment in so injudicious a manner is apt to bring a meritorious method into discredit. The first step of a successful treatment must, therefore, be a correct diagnosis, and this requires inspection through a speculum. It is high time that the traditional administration of vaginal douches be curtailed. Very little can be said in favor of them, as I have stated more in detail on page 317 of the original monograph. There is an occasional indication in purely vaginal discharge, but in cervical or corporeal leukorrhea the douche can accomplish nothing. Yet, it is no rarity to hear from patients that such douches had been prescribed for them four or more times a day!

The vaginitis due to trichomonas requires a specific treatment as described on page 211. The discharge of senile vaginitis will yield to the measures presented on page 168.

The sovereign remedy both for vaginal and cervical discharges is the powder treatment inaugurated by Nassauer. This method is fully discussed on page 349. Its efficacy may be gauged by the numerous imitations and modifications it has brought forth in recent years. I merely repeat here my recommendation to use equal parts of kaolin and bicarbonate of soda for the insufflations which are made every two or three days.

In obstinate cervical discharges, and particularly in cases where everted and eroded cervical lips keep up the irritation of the cervical mucosa, the powder treatment should be combined with electrocauterization according to the method of Dickinson which has been described fully on page 287. Since employing this combination of methods, I have been able to reduce the number of amputations of the cervix to a very large extent. The endlessly repeated cauterization of the cervix with tincture of iodin or silver nitrate which was a favorite method with the older generation of practitioners, is now definitely obsolete. One wonders whether the endurance of the patient was more to be admired or that of the physician!

Discharge from the endometrium itself presents an entirely different problem to the therapeutist. Each case demands individual study and treatment. The leukorrhea of young girls needs no local treatment but will yield to a general hygiene enforced, perhaps, by some iron and arsenic. In endocrine disturbances the corresponding organotherapeutic remedies, empirical and incomplete though they are, must be employed. Fibroids call for either radium or surgical measures, according to the principles laid down on page 134. Retroflexions may require orthopedic or surgical treatment; if the latter, a curettage may at times precede the operative cure of the displacement, *and this is the only instance where a curettage is permissible in the treatment of leukorrhea.* Subinvolution of long standing often necessitates a hysterectomy, but not infrequently a combination of glycerin tampons in the manner described on page 279, and protracted hot douches, discussed and depicted on pages 161 and 318, will give relief. Chronic infections of the uterus and its vicinity may yield to the same combination of treatment, particularly if supported by protein therapy, but, on the whole, radical surgical removal will give more satisfactory results.

To go into further details would be a repetition of much that has been said elsewhere in this book. The main purpose of these lines is to emphasize that leukorrhea is a symptom of a number of morbid processes and that its cure depends on an accurate differentiation and the proper selection of the therapeutic means at our disposal.

**Protein Therapy.**—Continued observation has confirmed in me the conviction of the fundamental and far-reaching value of protein therapy in inflammatory diseases of the female genitals. I have occasionally employed the pharmaceutical preparations of sterile milk in ampules, but, on the whole, I have seen no reason to discard the use of ordinary milk. The technic of preparation and injection has remained unaltered from the description given on page 342. Only one improvement has been added in the last few months. K. D. Graves, of Roanoke, suggested injections with centrifugalized and fat-free milk (*J. Am. M. Ass.*, 1924, 84:1505) and I can fully subscribe to his claim that such milk produces no local irritation; both the general and focal reactions are greatly reduced without any apparent influence on the efficacy of the procedure.

My own experiences which now extend over a period of almost four years and comprise many hundreds of injections, have recently been presented in an article in the *American Journal of Obstetrics and Gynecology*, November, 1924, and correspond closely with those laid down in Chapter XXII of my monograph and thus require no repetition. An interesting observation not yet recorded by me concerns a case of large bilateral pus tubes which subsided under milk injections. Some time later a laparotomy, performed for the relief of a retroflexion, revealed both tubes perfectly normal and patent. An identical case was reported to me by a friend and, in fact, I have received confirmations of my contentions of the value of milk injections from many quarters.

Where a simple and successful mode of treatment is employed widely, the danger of using it injudiciously looms large, and for this reason a plea for proper selection of cases and strict individualization of dose and interval is not out of place. It is not enough to point out the vast possibilities of this new therapy—its limitations, too, must be emphasized. There are several absolute contraindications, such as cardiac decompensation, diabetes, and alcoholism. Whether pregnancy belongs to this group, is still an open question. Petersen enjoins great caution where there is a history of hypersensitiveness on the part of the patient (serum sickness, asthma, urticaria, angioneurotic edema) or of epilepsy or other grave nervous instability. Above all, the state of the disease and the condition of the patient must be considered. Only if the cells are not hopelessly damaged or if the patient has not reached the state of complete fatigue, may milk injections be tried, lest they superimpose an extra demand to which the exhausted organism must succumb.

At no time should protein therapy be considered a cure-all; but even with all these restrictions and with all possible caution in the interpretation of the results achieved, protein therapy marks, to my mind, one of the greatest advances in therapeutics in recent times.

# COMPLICATIONS OF PREGNANCY

EDWARD P. DAVIS, M.D.

## APPENDIX

**The Late Hegar's Sign.**—Under this title attention has been called to the fact that Hegar's sign is present for some time after the uterus has been emptied in early pregnancy. If a vaginal examination be made at this time the lower segment is plainly evident, the cervix is soft but may have closed immediately after the expulsion of the embryo, so that practically it does not admit the examining finger. The shape, size and consistency of the uterus is that of early pregnancy. Under these circumstances it is impossible for a physician from one examination, to know whether the patient is at that time pregnant or whether an embryo has very recently escaped from the uterus. The patient must be put under accurate and continual observation for a number of weeks; during this time if the uterus grows smaller and gradually assumes its non-pregnant condition, it is fair to infer that it no longer contains, certainly, a living embryo. It is true that a blighted ovum may be retained in the uterus indefinitely, but a living embryo cannot be present without continual uterine growth.

Should a menstrual period develop, the diagnosis that the patient is not pregnant becomes clear.

Joachimovits (*Monatschr. f. Geburtsh. u. Gynaek.* Band 67, Heft 5, 1924) in his examination of 50 cases of abortion where the uterus was entirely emptied, found Hegar's sign clearly demonstrable in two cases, and present to some extent in 11 cases, five days after the escape of the ovum. There was slight hemorrhage in these patients but not sufficient to be of service in the matter of diagnosis.

That a dead fetus may be retained in the uterine cavity has long been known. Karlin (*Monatschr. f. Geburtsh. u. Gynaek.*, Band 67, Heft 5, 1924) reports three cases in one of which a dead fetus was retained in a woman suffering from carcinoma of the cervix, for one and one-half months from its death. Another woman with mitral lesion of the heart and toxemia, retained a fetus for a month after its death, while in a third case, a month after the death of the child stenosis of the internal os developed which made the emptying of the uterus difficult.

**Diagnosis of Pregnancy by the X-Ray.**—This means of diagnosis, so valuable in other branches of medicine, is of decided importance in pregnancy. Its success will depend, not only upon the ability and experience of the operator, but also upon the perfection of the instrument employed.

Under ordinary circumstances several months at least must have elapsed before an accurate picture showing fetal bones can be obtained. With the average x-ray five months is often as early as one can obtain accurate results, although under exceptional circumstances an earlier shadow develops.

The use of the x-ray to diagnosticate complications in pregnancy increases in value as time goes on. In a recent case of twin pregnancy, a positive diagnosis of the twin pregnancy was not clear. It was thought that one large child might be in the uterus or twins. The x-ray showed twin pregnancy but further demonstrated the fact that the twins were in such a position that should labor develop, they would inevitably become locked. The significance of this is apparent.

If one large child had been present, cesarean section was indicated as the pelvis was less than the average in size and the head had not engaged. If twins were present it was to be expected that as each twin is rarely of average size, vaginal delivery would readily occur; the presence of locked twins, however, in a primipara between 30 and 40 years of age, made cesarean section still the proper method of delivery.

**The Serological Diagnosis of Pregnancy.**—This still remains without satisfactory results. The Abderhalden test has long since been shown inaccurate. That disturbance of metabolism follows certain procedures in pregnancy which does not happen in the non-pregnant, is indirectly of some slight value, thus the injection of epinephrin in pregnant patients is followed by glycosuria. In pregnant patients the red blood corpuscles are said to settle to the bottom of a container much more rapidly than those of non-pregnant, but these are conditions which give rise to inference only and are of little value for positive information.

The metabolism of pregnancy remains an unsolved problem in the very extensive and increasing literature. The fact that pregnant women lose in weight is of interest and various researches have been made upon this point. In a recent series of observations by Hirsch (*Monatschr. f. Geburtsh. u. Gynaek.*, Band 67, Heft. 5, 1924) in 170 pregnant patients, 53.5 per cent were below the average weight. The patients under observation for some time in the hospital, showed that there was a slight gain in weight until the sixth day before labor, from this to the fourth day the weight remained unchanged, and then occurred a loss so that when labor began, the average weight was 0.4 kilograms less than five days before labor. It is difficult to find an explanation of this fact, but it may be of interest to note that the x-ray applied to the hypophysis in some patients produces a loss of weight.

An observation of some interest in this connection is made by Hess and Weinstock (*J. Am. M. Ass.*, Nov. 15, 1924) concerning the influence exerted by the diet of a pregnant woman, upon rickets in her offspring. By experiment upon animals the writers found that giving cod-liver oil during pregnancy did not protect the fetus against rickets when after birth the young were placed under conditions favorable for the production of rickets. At the Sloane Hospital for Women a number of pregnant patients were given cod-liver oil during the last two months of pregnancy; 28 patients could be observed and of this number, 15 had infants which developed rickets according to clinical criteria and eight of these were shown to have rickets by x-ray examination.

That the mother's nutrition has an influence in making the child susceptible to rickets is proved by the fact that premature infants are very susceptible to the development of the disease. Evidently the nutrition of the mother in pregnancy has little to do with the disease in the child and this is acquired after its birth.

**Metabolism of the Pregnant Woman as Regards the Development of Eclampsia.**—This is studied by Monahert (*Arch. f. Gynæk.*, 1923, 119:407). His paper is devoted largely to the question of oxidation. Carbohydrates are less oxidized in the pregnant than in the non-pregnant, so are protein substances. While as regards the fetus the absorption of oxygen is increased and the passage of carbon dioxid is less in proportion to the quantity taken. Of the nitrogenous substances taken by the pregnant woman there is less oxidation than in the non-pregnant. As toxemia increases, so does carbon dioxid in direct ratio to the severity of the complication. Acid compounds are formed and if the kidneys become considerably affected the complication is more severe. The injection of adrenalin in pregnant patients increases metabolism but less than in the non-pregnant; there was a secondary increase followed by a decided drop in the non-pregnant. Less oxygen is absorbed and less carbon dioxid excreted after adrenalin is taken. There is some relation between blood pressure and oxidation in the body of the pregnant woman, there seems to be retention in the venous blood in the pregnant woman of carbon dioxid resulting from some degree of acidosis. In toxemic patients the alkalescence of the blood is often materially lessened; while this process has to do with the growth of the fetus it often indicates an abnormal condition of the mother. In 57 per cent of patients suffering from derangement in function of the thyroid, this condition could be demonstrated by chemical studies in the metabolism. Knaus (*Arch. f. Gynæk.*, 1923, 119:450) reviews the function of the thyroid in pregnancy by calling attention to hypothyroidism with lessened secretion, accumulation of partially formed substances, high content of globulin poor in iodin, with lessened quantity of cellular thyroid globulin rich in iodin. In contrast to this is hyperthyroidism having increased secretion, an accumulation of imperfectly formed material diminished in globulin and its iodin, and increase of iodin which contains globulin showing a lack of colloid material. This lack of colloid substances is invariably present when the thyroid is deranged in its action in pregnancy, although pregnancy causes the colloid to increase in quantity, its content is poor in iodin and so its function of efficiency is lessened. During the last half of pregnancy the mother stores up nitrogen which has been estimated as four times the quantity absolutely necessary for the growth of the fetus. Undoubtedly the development of the breasts is concerned in this. When myxedema and cretinism develop in pregnancy, hypothyroidism becomes extreme. When pregnancy develops in women from whom the greater part of the thyroid has been removed, a condition analogous to tetany often develops.

**The Respiratory Function in Pregnancy.**—This was studied by Bombani (*Ann. d'obst.*, 1923, 10:528) in a nervous pregnant woman who had influenza in 1918 and at four months pregnancy had obstinate and severe dyspnea. The urine was negative, the blood normal and abdominal organs seemed healthy.

There was some tendency to exophthalmos but the pupils reacted well. The blood showed over four million red cells and 7000 white cells and 75 per cent hemoglobin. Various drugs were given to the patient and the carbon dioxid content was studied. While some of the observations are interesting, they throw no definite light upon the problem.

The question has often arisen as to whether *osteomalacia* is a disease congenital in the pregnant woman and only requiring pregnancy for its development, or whether it is acquired. In *Surgery, Gynecology and Obstetrics,* November, 1924, Stone reviews the literature of the subject, adding his own researches which go to show that the disease is acquired. The exact cause is at present unknown and there is no direct proof that endocrines are responsible for the disease. It is known that calcium is deficient in the blood of these patients and yet very little attention has been paid to the condition of the parathyroid in these cases. The two substances which seem to be lacking in the mother's nutrition are cod-liver oil and vitamin A.

Researches by Dragstedt call attention to the connection between the parathyroid and metabolism in pregnant animals.

The influence of work on the pregnant woman is of interest not only for general consideration concerning the success of pregnancy, but also with regard to the possible development of the toxemia of pregnancy. Carlinir (*Rev. franç. d'obst.,* 1923, 19), reviews extensively the literature upon the subject. There is no question that rest for the mother in the last weeks of pregnancy secures a better condition for her and the better development of the child. This rest does not exclude moderate and healthy exercise.

In contrast to this is the effect produced by painful and excessive work, especially if carried on under unfavorable hygienic conditions. Women working in shops, factories, and arsenals are naturally under more unfavorable conditions than those working in the country, their nutrition is worse and so is that of the offspring. Many pregnant women cannot work in tobacco factories without suffering. Painful and excessive work in a mother, especially if done in an uncomfortable and cramped posture, may shorten pregnancy, bringing the patient into premature labor. Unquestionably abortion is more common among women engaged in work than among those who are not, but this is not so much the result of the fact that these women work, as depending upon the circumstances that make them work under unfavorable conditions and injuriously.

New light is given to our study of the *Relation of the Embryo and the Mother,* by Teacher (*J. Obst. & Gynæc. Brit. Emp.,* 1924, 31, 2). This contains some exceedingly good and clear illustrations, showing the intimate relation between the villi of the chorion and the maternal blood, and also the relation of the maternal blood to the ovum before the intervillous spaces are formed. His study shows a remarkable connection between the blood of the mother and the embryo which must render the condition of the mother's blood a potent factor in influencing her offspring.

The effect has been made to show the *Relationship between the Area of Placental Attachment and the Birth Weight of the Child* by Lavake (*Am. J. Obst.,* July, 1924). He concludes from his study of the subject that the diet of the mother influences little or not at all the size of the child, it is therefore useless to limit the diet in the mother to lessen the fetal size or to push her nourishment excessively with the hope of stimulating the growth of the embryo.

The toxemia of pregnancy is always a subject fertile in literary production. Many obstetricians believe that the toxemia of pregnancy is essentially one process, differing in manifestation in different organs and under different circumstances. This view seems logical and is useful in presenting the matter to students for study.

Some, however, strongly dissent from this opinion, among them Cook (*Brit. M. J.*, March 1924 in the *Hunterian Lecture on the Toxemia of Pregnancy*). His contention is essentially that until toxemias are clearly recognized, demonstrated and analyzed, he declines to believe that they exist as decisive factors in what is termed by some the toxemia of pregnancy. He questions the variations from the normal which are alleged to exist in calcium content of the blood serum in pregnancy, and he does not accept the findings of those who have detected in the blood serum marked variations in the healthy pregnant patient and in those threatened with eclampsia, having albuminuria or who have eclampsia.

The acidosis factor he believes of little importance and in eclampsia the inorganic constituents are very little changed. Biochemical investigations have given us no accurate knowledge. The average case of albuminuria he asserts shows no symptoms. He believes that mechanical pressure of the growing uterus interferes with the function of some of the excretory organs. The value of bleeding in toxemia is its effect upon blood pressure. The pernicious nausea of gestation is caused by many factors among which starvation is very important. The influence of the nervous system is paramount, and he would not withhold food from these patients.

The majority of evidence, however, does not support his contention that there are no essential alterations in the blood urea and in the metabolic processes of the mother who has toxemia. It has been thought that in many cases of toxemia of gestation, the death of the fetus in utero is favorable for the mother. Recent studies in this connection indicate that where the fetus dies in the uterus and the mother's toxemic condition immediately grows less, the woman has no definite lesion of the excretory organs, especially the kidneys; but if albuminuria and other signs of toxemia persist after the death of the fetus, structural changes have developed in the excretory organs.

*The Condition of the Eye in the Pregnant Toxemic Patient* is always interesting, and Cheyney (*J. Am. M. Ass.*, Nov., 1924) reports his experience in examining patients at the Boston Lying-in Hospital. He found that retinitis complicating pregnancy is not more common in primiparæ than in multiparæ. When changes occur in the fundus they usually develop in the last three months of pregnancy but rarely recur. If the toxemia of pregnancy is acute, eye changes do not recur; but if the pregnant woman has chronic nephritis, eye changes persist and return often with increased severity, in subsequent pregnancy.

In 8400 patients in the Clinic at Christiania were 680 whose eyes were examined and among these were 40 cases of retinitis; 82 per cent of patients with retinitis had chronic nephritis and 18 had an acute toxemia of pregnancy. The reports of different observers do not agree concerning the permanent damage to vision. In one series, but 65 per cent of patients having retinitis were able to read after the pregnancy had ended. In another series 28 per cent had normal vision, 58 per cent damaged vision, and 14 per cent were blind after pregnancy ended. The writer believes that if a toxemic patient shows retinitis the chances are 4 to 1 that she had developed kidney lesions and she should be carefully followed for over a year after the termination of pregnancy. Unless the urine and blood pressure are absolutely normal during this time, repeated pregnancy must not occur. It is true that cases of chronic nephritis can be tided along for considerable periods, and with these patients retinitis processes as well; but this does not lessen the gravity of the situation.

So far as treatment is concerned, if retinitis is discovered at any time previous to the last two weeks of pregnancy, the pregnancy should be terminated. Patients having retinitis and going to term, show a mortality of 15 per cent, and 20 per cent blindness in the survivors. Where the pregnancy is interrupted, the mortality falls to 4 per cent and the percentage of blindness to 6 per cent. Retinitis may be caused by toxic blood or may be secondary to changes in the circulatory system such as increased blood pressure, slowing of the circulation, and hemorrhage.

In studying pregnant patients the writer endeavored to ascertain whether by examination of the eyes he could distinguish an acute toxemic case from the nephritic. Where the condition was one of acute toxemia it should theoretically be easy to differentiate from chronic nephritis, but practically it is impossible to do so, for lesions in the retina may vary in character, extent, and development in both toxemia and nephritic patients.

That it is important to have the eyes of pregnant patients examined, there can be no doubt and in many cases a valuable indication of the toxemia of pregnancy may thus be found. In the writer's observation the spontaneous interruption of pregnancy in these cases is often a conservative process not only to save the life of the mother but frequently to preserve her vision.

*Toxemia of Pregnancy as a Cause of Mental Disease.*—That the toxemia of pregnancy is the cause of mental disease is demonstrated by Bourne (*J. Obst. & Gynæc. Brit. Emp.*, 1924, 31, 2). He was able to study with a fair degree of accuracy 61 cases of insanity. The two great causes of this condition are the toxemia of pregnancy and septic infection. It is interesting to note that patients having eclampsia usually recover more rapidly and often more completely, than those who had toxemia which did not end in eclampsia. This is also true as regard the mortality, the mortality of eclamptic patients is less than that of toxemic cases in which convulsions do not occur. Seventy-seven per cent of eclamptic patients had insanity for a short period after pregnancy terminated and then recovered their mental health. In cases, however, where the toxemia did not clear up, repeated pregnancy was accompanied by repeated attacks of insanity.

At the Bellevue Hospital, Gregory (*Am. J. Obst.*, Oct. 1924) studied 118 cases of mental disease complicating parturition. More than half were called manic depressive psychoses. This is stated to be a constitutional disorder with a definite history and usually terminated favorably.

*That sudden death after labor is due to a degenerative condition of the liver and a severe toxemia* is illustrated by the report by Schickele (*Gynécologie et Obstétrique,* 1924, 1) in his clinic at Strassburg. His first patient was aged 35, second pregnancy, spontaneous labor followed by some hemorrhage and manual removal of the placenta. There had been very moderäte anesthesia with ether. After delivery the patient became greatly cyanosed and died in an hour. At autopsy the liver was extensively disintegrated and necrotic. Kidney lesions were not important.

The second patient was a young woman in labor 15 hours, delivered by low forceps application, the child was living and vigorous but the mother died four hours after labor. Autopsy revealed an extensive lesion of the liver with embolism, no lesions in the heart or other organs. The liver was extensively disintegrated. On examination the capillaries were dilated and there was multiple hemorrhage and various stages of cellular degeneration. The kidney lesions were very slight.

A third case was in her fourth pregnancy with rachitic pelvis. Cesarean section under spinal anesthesia was done. Just after the child was delivered, the patient became livid, respiration failed, and death ensued. The spinal anesthesia was considered as the cause of death. At autopsy the liver showed lesions of yellow atrophy.

*The Toxemia of Pregnancy with Especial Reference to Liver Function* was studied by Berkeley and his associates, as reported in the *J. Obst. & Gynæc. Brit. Emp.,* 1924, 31, 1. He examined cases from a number of hospitals and completed his paper by tables and statistics. He was especially interested in two methods of research: one the estimation of the blood urea and blood non-protein nitrogen; the other the investigation of the urine. In another group of investigations which he found more important, were the tests of hepatic function. For this purpose he used Fouchet's test for bile pigment in the blood. This is based upon the circumstance that damage to the liver cells causes them to lose the property of converting urobilin into bile pigments; urobilin then accumulates in the blood and is excreted in the urine and can be recognized. Fouchet's test consists in taking the serum of the patient examined, putting three drops on a white porcelain surface and adding three drops of the reagent employed. This reagent is 20 c.c. $H_2O$, 2 c.c. of 10 per cent ferric chlorid, 5 Gms. trichloracetic acid. If the reaction is positive, a white coagulum is formed by precipitation of the serum proteids by the trichloracetic acid and the coagulum turns a greenish blue color, reaching a maximum in about twenty minutes. He employed other tests but Fouchet's he believed was of considerable importance.

This paper should be studied in detail by those especially interested in the toxemia of pregnancy.

The purpose of the study was to determine whether an indication could be found which would form a reliable guide for the interruption of pregnancy and it is believed that the best indication and perhaps the only safe one for inducing premature labor in cases of albuminuria of pregnancy, is the test of hepatic function described. Even if the blood urea and non-protein nitrogen tests are as reliable as they are considered, they are complicated, requiring expensive apparatus and high technical skill, while Fouchet's test is simple and can be readily applied.

In line with this investigation is the report of a case of pernicious nausea of pregnancy with acidosis, treated by insulin. (Lequeux. *Bull. Soc. d'obst.*, 1924, 5). The patient was aged 29, good general health. Eight months after marriage she had some treatment for the pelvic organs and after that pregnancy developed. Pernicious nausea was present with very great tenderness over the abdomen. Apparently menstruation returned and an early abortion had probably taken place. The second pregnancy was followed by pernicious nausea with severe acidosis, the coefficient being 68 per cent and acetone abundantly present in the urine. Treatment by injections of adrenalin and suprarenal extract did little or no good. Glucose was given by rectum. This treatment seemed to be successful for some time when the patient again became worse and was again better with the treatment. She gave birth to a child deficient in weight but made a recovery. In the next pregnancy nausea was treated by ovarian extract successfully with the successful termination of pregnancy. In a following pregnancy pernicious nausea was again present and the patient was treated by the administration of glucose and the Lily preparation of 10 units of insulin. She grew better, then worse, but her physicians were able to carry her along in pregnancy until a uterine hemorrhage occurred. A dilating bag was then placed in the uterus and under anesthesia a living child delivered by version.

In a recent number of the *Journal of the American Medical Association*, Thalhimer reports his experience with glucose and insulin in the pernicious nausea of early pregnancy. He gives by intravenous injection 1000 c.c. of 10 per cent pure glucose and also 10 units of insulin are administered. This treatment was repeated in these proportions three times in severe cases with good results. His series of cases would aggregate a considerable number.

In a case of pernicious nausea and toxemia at about seven months pregnancy in a multipara who had had toxemia in each of five previous pregnancies, the writer employed the intravenous glucose and insulin treatment. The uterus expelled its contents in this case. The first administration of glucose and insulin was followed by improvement, the second was followed in a few hours by high fever, coma, and death. Autopsy showed degenerative changes in the liver and kidneys.

**Syphilis in Pregnancy.**—The question of syphilis in pregnancy remains, as always, of great importance. In a paper in the *British Medical Journal*, November, 1923, Roberts states that in England and Wales, 10 per cent of all marriages are complicated by syphilis and in these families three-quarters of the children are infected and one-third of the pregnancies end in fetal death. If syphilitic children are born alive, three-quarters die in the first year and the mortality later is very high.

In diagnosis the Wassermann reaction is of value but it is not absolutely conclusive. In seven-eighths of the cases a positive Wassermann in the mother means syphilis during pregnancy. So far as the period of pregnancy in which infection is most fatal for the child is concerned, if the mother becomes syphilitic before the end of the fifth month, the child does not escape; at the fifth or sixth month, there is 50 per cent chance for fetal mortality or fetal life, but if the mother contracts syphilis after the seventh month of pregnancy, the child escapes. The earlier in the pregnancy the mother is infected the more likely is the pregnancy to be interrupted. Multiparæ resist infection better than primiparæ.

Syphilitic pregnant women suffer considerably from headache, neuralgia, and insomnia, which are more or less relieved by appropriate treatment. During pregnancy, for primary and secondary signs, prompt treatment should be instituted. If a clinical diagnosis of syphilis can be made, no matter what the Wassermann reaction is, the mother should receive arsphenamin. If the disease is latent, neoarsphenamin should be given in weekly injections increasing to the twenty-eighth day, then ceasing for a week while other remedies are given. During this treatment the urine should be frequently examined to detect irritation of the kidneys. Pain should be avoided and the patient's teeth should be cared for. The dosage in this treatment is .03 grn. in the beginning increased to .06 grn., the treatment stopping for a week every three or four weeks. During the entire time of treatment 1 grn. of mercury in chalk should be taken three times daily, and from 7 to 10 grns. of potassium iodid three times daily from the tenth to the twelfth and twenty-sixth to the twenty-eighth week.

*The Wassermann Reaction* was studied at the Edinburgh Royal Maternity Hospital; Browne (*J. Obst. & Gynæc. Brit. Emp.*, 1923, 4) found that in old syphilis the only evidence obtainable during pregnancy was the Wassermann reaction in 75 per cent of cases. Primiparæ did not resist infection as well as multiparæ, which has been shown by other observers.

There was no definite evidence that the Wassermann reaction is changed to any great degree by pregnancy. In a suspicious case both parents should be under observation during pregnancy with repeated Wassermann tests in the mother.

Klaften (*Zentralbl. f. Gynäk.* 1924, 35) reports the results of his studies in the diagnosis of syphilis in parturient women by examining retroplacental blood at the time of labor. This was found to be a more delicate and certain test than the Wassermann reaction in the blood taken from a vein. Extract diluted 8 to 12 times was used; 0.4 c.cm. of retroplacental blood serum was mixed with 1 c.c. (1 to 11) with 2 per cent salt solution and the mixture was warmed. In from four to twenty-four hours the fluid became clotted and cloudy. This was produced by the increase in the colloids and the proteid bodies of the blood serum. By this accurate chemical observation a considerable number of cases of latent syphilis were discovered which otherwise would not have been detected.

In cases of abortion in early pregnancy, about 10 per cent gave a positive serum reaction. It is important to note whether syphilis is present in a parturient woman before delivery, especially in recognizing accurately the cause of fetal death should the child perish during a difficult delivery. The operation may be blamed for the death, but if the mother was syphilitic during pregnancy, autopsy will frequently show that the child was syphilitic and that the real cause of infant death was syphilis in the mother; also the presence of syphilis may complicate her recovery from abdominal section.

*The Treatment of Parturient Patients by Sera and Such Remedies as Arsphenamin* must not be employed without reference to the interests of the child. It is known that the treatment of syphilis in the mother may influence the child unfavorably in some cases. That vaccines may injure the child when given to the mother is shown by Fischer (*Zentralbl. f. Gynäk.* 1924, 40), who gave a vaccine to a pregnant woman suffering from pyelitis. On the sixth day afterward she had a severe urticaria eruption on the thighs and buttocks, the throat and tonsils were red and swollen, the cervical glands enlarged, and the throat became so swollen that it was feared tracheotomy would be necessary. The eruption spread over the whole body, spontaneous labor developed, and abundant hemorrhages were found in the body of the dead child. There was no evidence of syphilis.

He cites other cases of pyelitis where the use of vaccines was followed by fetal death.

**Pyelitis in Pregnancy.**—PYELITIS STILL REMAINS A NOT INFREQUENT, ANNOYING, AND SOMETIMES DANGEROUS COMPLICATION OF PREGNANCY. Klaften (*Zentralbl. f. Gynäk.*, 1924, 32) divides his cases into three groups: (1) Those who recovered apparently perfectly; 50 per cent of his patients were in this class. (2) The patient recovered so far as symptoms of illness were concerned but the urine remained cloudy containing leucocytes and bacillus colicommunis in pure culture. This condition persisted indefinitely in some cases. (3) In the third group the patient passed through pregnancy and labor and seemed to improve very rapidly, but the urine persisted in an abnormal condition indefinitely, containing colon bacilli and other germs. These patients seemed to have latent pyelitis as part of their general condition. Such patients may be called "carriers" as the urine is distinctly infectious.

This disease occurs about equally in primiparæ and multiparæ and diagnosis is sometimes difficult because the signs and symptoms, when the pyelitis is in the right kidney, resemble those of appendicitis, and cases are cited in which pyelitis very closely simulated typhoid infection. In differential diagnosis it is useful to examine the vaginal secretion where the colon bacillus is found in great numbers and various forms. They are usually absent in the upper third of the vagina and under ordinary circumstances the colon bacillus is destroyed by the normal vaginal secretion in forty-eight hours. Where, however, the vaginal secretion becomes pathological, the colon bacilli survive ten days or longer. Vaginal douches of lactic acid are often useful in these cases.

So far as the cause of the condition is concerned constipation and obstruction of the ureters are the principal factors. It is rare to find cystitis and pyelitis combined in these patients. Mild cases of this sort yield readily to treatment but severe cases are difficult to manage and dangerous. Urotropin is useful, and fatal cases result from suppurating infarcts in the kidneys. It must also be remembered that some of these cases date their pyelitis to an attack of this condition in childhood, which was very probably not detected;

after severe scarlatina or measles the child may be left with a chronic condition which so long as the general health is good, escapes observation.

The majority of obstetricians have treated these cases conservatively: rest in bed, careful diet, urotropin, whose action is increased, it is thought, by giving dilute hydrochloric acid at the same time, vaginal douches of lactic acid, and mild purgation were the remedies most employed. Irrigation of the pelvis of the kidney is valuable in severe cases, but without other treatment it will not relieve the severe cases. Fifty per cent of these patients make a complete recovery with judicious treatment.

**Eclampsia.**—The treatment of eclampsia is the source of unending discussion and gradually material of interest is acquired from the vast accounts which this serious complication of pregnancy produces. The Stroganoff treatment remains a subject of frequent discussion.

At a meeting of the Section of Obstetrics and Gynecology of the Royal Society of Medicine, London, Stroganoff presented a paper upon this subject (*Brit. M. J.*, July 12, 1924). He alludes to the high mortality produced by eclampsia, then claims that a universal application of his method of treatment would reduce this at least one half. His method was first employed in 1897 in 57 cases without a death. In 1918, 2208 cases treated by this method, collected from the literature, showed a maternal mortality of 9.8 per cent. In 1924, 3302 cases had been so treated with a mortality of 10.8 per cent. In his own observation and treatment, in ten years there had been six deaths, 2.4 per cent, and of these deaths three were from other causes. Not only was death made less common, but the patients were less severely ill and complications were greatly reduced. Psychic disturbances occurred in only 1.6 per cent; fetal mortality was reduced to 14.3 per cent.

He repeated the details of his treatment as follows: The removal of all sources of possible irritation, a darkened room, oxygen for asphyxia, careful protection during the convulsion, one-sixth grain morphin hypodermically injected, followed one hour later by 30 grns. chloral hydrate by mouth or rectum. Two hours later the morphin is repeated, four hours after this the chloral, 20 grns. of chloral is given 13 and 21 hours after the beginning of the treatment. If the child is still undelivered at the end of 24 hours, 14 to 20 grns. of chloral should be given three times a day. If, in spite of this, convulsions occur, 400 c.c. of blood should be taken from a vein. If labor comes on, delivery of the child should be aided. The functions of the body should be promoted as far as possible. Hot bottles should be placed about the patient and warm fluids should be taken freely. The patient is kept on her right side, the mouth is carefully cleansed and oxygen is given for asphyxia. If the pulse reaches 110 or more, digitalis is administered with camphor or caffein. Bleeding was practiced in 10 per cent of cases and then only if three or more fits occurred after the treatment was commenced. If it was thought that the patient could be delivered within two hours, bleeding was not practiced.

**Inflammation of the Uterine Adnexa Complicating Pregnancy.**—While comparatively rare, this is frequently a serious condition. Patients with chronic inflammation of the tubes and ovaries are usually sterile. In other cases, however, there has been partial recovery and then pregnancy supervenes.

Some of these have tubal pregnancy, others have pregnancy with more or less active inflammation of the fallopian tubes, varying in severity. These cases usually result from gonorrhea. A hematogenic infection with the pregnancy is often located in the corpus luteum and the primary focus is frequently in the tonsils or some other part of the organism abounding in bacteria. Appendicitis during pregnancy may cause infection of the adjacent fallopian tube and result in local peritonitis. From the anatomy of pregnancy, the ascending form of infection in the fallopian tube must be rare; it can develop only during the early months before the deciduous membranes have joined. These cases arise from gonorrhea and often end in abortion. Attempts at criminal abortion frequently result in a purulent salpingitis. In these cases an abscess may rupture during pregnancy and be followed by a rapidly fatal peritonitis and sepsis.

There are abundant reports of cases in which foreign bodies have been introduced into the uterus to interrupt pregnancy and have perforated the uterus and been removed from the abdomen.

When an infection or injury is not severe, pregnant patients may recover without abortion. Very rarely the pregnancy causes a previous condition of inflammation in the pelvic organs to disappear. If adhesions are present in the pelvis, the result of pregnancy may be disastrous. Labor may rupture an abscess causing infection.

Schmid (*Arch. f. Gynæk.*, 1923, 120:31) reports four fatal cases complicating pregnancy where foci of infection in the pelvis ruptured.

There are a number of reports showing the development of primary chorionepithelioma of the broad ligament complicating pregnancy. The disease may also attack the ovary and a diagnosis cannot be positively made until tissue can be removed at operation. All patients in whom, during or immediately after the pregnancy, suspicious symptoms arise, calling attention to the possibility of this condition, should be subjected to thorough study and operation for the examination of tissues. Realizing that the condition is hopeless if pronounced, no delay should be practiced in suspicious cases. It must be remembered that this condition develops only after pregnancy or during pregnancy, and that it is one of the most dangerous results of pregnancy.

That chorionepithelioma of the ovary is rare, is shown by Dougal (*J. Obst. & Gynæc. Brit. Emp.*, 1924, 31, 3), who with his own, collected, in the literature, 11 cases.

In some respects resembling this is **ileus,** complicating pregnancy. These cases are seen in constipated pregnant patients, and a diagnosis is often more readily obtained by examination with the x-ray. This shows the intestines greatly distended and may indicate a point of occlusion. The diagnosis is made in the usual manner with operation promptly performed as the only efficient method of treating these cases.

**Cancer of the stomach** complicating pregnancy, while not a very frequent occurrence, is, like cancer, at any time exceedingly grave as a condition. Schmid (*Arch. f. Gynæk.*, Band 121, Heft 2, 1924) studied 44 cases, in 14 of which there was metastasis in the fallopian tubes. The children were lost in two-thirds of these cases and the writer could not trace a single permanent recovery in the mother. Obviously if this condition can be recognized, immediate operation is imperative.

Experiments on animals seemed to indicate that the effort to inoculate pregnant animals with malignant growths is less successful than in the non-pregnant.

**Cancer of the neck of the uterus** complicating pregnancy, would at present naturally suggest the use of radium or x-ray in treatment. Complete recovery is reported by Couvelier (*Gynéc. & Obst.*, 1924, 2) in the seventh pregnancy of a woman aged 35. This patient came into labor, was delivered by section followed by supravaginal hysterectomy, and application of radium to the cancerous cervix by the abdominal route. The child was living when delivered. With the aid of a special trocar, four tubes of radium were placed in the cervix, one in front, one behind, one on the right and one on the left, each tube containing 10 Mgms. of radium element with a filter of 1 mm. of platinum. A bag was placed in Douglas' culdesac and also in the vesico-uterine pouch. Five days later the radium was removed from the abdomen and an application made in the vagina. The bags were gradually removed and the radium changed, its application being continued in all for 11 days and two-thirds of the radium being given by the abdominal route and one-third by the vaginal route. The patient made a complete recovery.

An interesting question arises as to child-bearing after radium and x-ray treatment. If this treatment is employed, what are the chances of pregnancy afterward? Pemberton reviews the literature of the subject and reports cases from Graves' Clinic in Boston (*Surg., Gynec. & Obst.*, Aug. 1924). Observation shows that the action of radium and x-ray is essentially the same. The maturing graafian follicles are more susceptible to radiation than the primordial, and radiation causes degeneration and destruction of the ovum preventing the follicle from coming to maturity and leaving a small cyst. If the follicle is not advanced the ovum is destroyed and a single layer of granulosa cells remains. Such a dose of radium may be used that mature follicles are destroyed and the primordial follicles are not damaged. We have no information concerning the possibility of fertilization of the partially damaged ovum, whether this would result in the formation of a poorly developed child or a deformed child is not known. Women treated by irradiation have a larger percentage of abortions than those who are not. In cold blooded animals radium and x-ray have produced malformations and lack of development. This has been observed in guinea pigs and there are a few reports of similar cases in human beings.

In the Munich Clinic, Werner, in 1500 cases treated by radiation traced 24 pregnancies with 13 well developed normal children, one premature, 9 abortions, and a hysterectomy for fibroids. Six of the pregnancies occurred in patients who had amenorrhea for several months after the treatment. All of these women showed diminished menstruation. There was one abortion to every two normal births. Others report normal children born whose mothers had been treated by radium. In one case where pregnancy was not recognized, radium was placed in the vagina for treatment and the child was small and backward in physical development when 3½ years old. A mother was x-rayed from the third to the sixth month of pregnancy on mistaken diagnosis of fibromyoma. The child was a microcephalic imbecile with atrophy and cloudiness of the lens of the eye. This same condition had been produced in animals by experiment.

Pemberton reports four cases of women who had been treated by radium and who afterward became pregnant. One had twins, one of whom died; the other survived and was well when 2½ years old. One had had no pregnancy before radiation but afterward gave birth to a normal child. One had eight children and after radium treatment became pregnant, with eclampsia and premature birth, the child living two days. Another was treated by radium for membranous dysmenorrhea. When pregnancy occurred she had an abortion at three months.

Attention is called to the severe **anemia** often accompanying the toxemic conditions in pregnancy by Schneider (*Monatschr. f. Geburtsh. u. Gynæk.*, Band 65, Heft 6, 1924). It has long been known that hemolysis may result in these cases and may be so severe as to become rapidly fatal.

That **acetonemia** may threaten death to a pregnant woman has been shown by numerous reports on the subject of the toxemia of gestation. Rowland (*Bull. Soc. d'obst.*, 4, 1924) reviews the literature of the subject and reports a case in detail in which the patient had a very severe toxemia resembling encephalitis lethargica in which acetone seemed to be the principal agent. The interruption of pregnancy was successful in this case in rescuing the mother.

**Tuberculous Infection of the Lung.**—The interruption of pregnancy with sterilization is not infrequently practiced for severe tubercular infection of the lung complicating pregnancy. It is not always possible, however, to obtain statistics as to the permanent results of the total removal of the uterus and adnexa in advanced tuberculosis. Misgeld reports from Bumm's Clinic (*Zentralbl. f. Gynäk.*, 20, 1924) 56 cases. The patients selected were those who had no cavities in the lungs, were not neurotic and pregnancy not beyond the fourth month, for after the sixth month interruption or total extirpation was not thought indicated; these patients had already given birth to living children.

The results were 16 deaths, 28.2 per cent; 32 improved, 57.1 per cent; three were worse, 5.36 per cent; and two were neither better nor worse, 3.57 per cent. The operation consisted in the entire removal of the uterus and its adnexa. These cases are compared with 45 cases in which pregnancy was terminated by dilatation and curetting only. The comparison is interesting.

After total extirpation the mortality was 28.2 per cent; after curetting only, the mortality was 37.7 per cent; 57.1 per cent were improved after radical operation and none were improved where pregnancy was terminated by curetting. In two, 3.57 per cent, the tubercular disease was brought to a temporary cessation after the radical operation; after curetting 1.7 per cent seemed to be better. Of those who grew rapidly worse after total extirpation, there were 3, or 3.36 per cent, and after curetting, 16, or 45.5 per cent, in a series of 34 patients operated upon. Four, or 25 per cent, had severe nervous symptoms of the last 20 patients operated upon, but these symptoms were not such as to forbid recovery.

Thalhimer (*Surg., Gynec. & Obst.*, Aug., 1924) gives the results of some recent researches in the laboratory of the Columbia Hospital of Milwaukee in the *Insulin Treatment of the Toxemic Vomiting of Pregnancy.* He quotes three successful cases under the care of physicians other than himself and all these showed marked ketonuria and one had acidosis with carbon hydrate combining power of the blood plasma of 35. Three hours after an intravenous infusion of glucose and insulin, the blood plasma combining power was 48 and nineteen hours later 69. Insulin forces the body to oxidize to the utmost glucose and this results in consuming the products of incomplete fat metabolism; the ketonuria is thus lessened and reduced. The blood plasma carbon dioxid combining power is raised, acidosis ceases, and the patient improves. A diet rich in carbohydrates is then given. That pregnancy causes an abnormality in carbohydrate metabolism, the writer believes is clearly shown. The results of treatment are that the patient's urine is free of acetone in one or two hours and the alkali reserve raises about ten points. An excessive amount of acetone reappears in the urine in eighteen to twenty-four hours, but unless the patient becomes worse, it may be disregarded. Carbohydrate food should be administered but no fat and plenty of fluid. After vomiting has ceased for twenty-four hours, the patient may take any food desired except fat, and the carbohydrates should be in abundance. The blood should be examined at least twice.

One patient only had an insulin reaction and she responded immediately when 3 mms. of adrenalin were given hypodermically and two glasses of milk were administered by the mouth.

Thalhimer's method of preparing the glucose is described and the apparatus for administration is reproduced in an illustration.

A review in general of the *Treatment of Complications of Pregnancy,* is contributed by Aschner (*Arch. f. Gynæk.*, 1923, Band 120, Heft 96). He calls attention to the frequent occurrence of interstitial hemorrhage in the nervous system, the ear, respiratory tract, the digestive tract, kidneys, heart, blood vessels, bones, joints, and skin. He also stated that during pregnancy septic inflammation, catarrhal inflammation, and exudate are observed. Patients frequently complain of the first symptoms of a developing inflammation such as congestion, disturbance of sensation of the hands and feet, heaviness in the limbs, aching pain about the head and teeth, neuralgia, catarrh, hyperacidity, and constipation. Many suppose that these occur inevitably in all pregnancies and pay no attention to them. They are, however, important and are usually controlled by rest, carefully regulated diet, and the giving of alkalies.

The writer ascribes these symptoms to the influence of the fetus and decidua on maternal blood. Toxins are produced, some of which may be used in fetal growth but most of which are distinctly harmful. These symptoms are important as indicating the first stage of toxemia because at that stage patients yield readily to treatment.

There is also a tendency in all pregnant women to thrombosis, embolism, and their results, and to failure in the normal action of the heart with congestion in various organs, notably the kidneys, and in severe cases the development of eclampsia.

Unquestionably the ancient belief that pregnant patients would be benefited by losing blood, has some foundation in truth. Because of her plethoric condition the pregnant woman is more liable to infection, and when this occurs, it readily becomes severe. In the treatment of this condition elimination is of primary importance. Nothing compares in value with this method of treatment. That the condition is widespread and profound is shown by recent microscopic studies which demonstrate the fact that the capillaries are involved and that in blood-making organs this capillary involvement readily predisposes to disease.

In women of very dark complexion with a tendency to sluggish action of the liver, and abnormal condition of the blood, one sometimes observes the death of the child at a normal termination of pregnancy although the mother may be free from syphilis. In some cases she is very syphilitic. When no other cause can be found the death of the child must be due to a disturbance or failure in internal secretion in either the mother or the child. A considerable number of these mothers show hyperthyroidism and the greater number of children are males. To prevent such loss the fetal heart sounds should be watched, especially during labor and if they show signs of failure the child must be promptly delivered.

While an effort has been made to demonstrate a distinct pathological relation between the blood of the mother and child, this effort has so far not been successful.

The study of the blood in pregnant women is interesting and in 200 patients, in 44 primiparæ the average leucocyte count was 11,480; while in multiparæ it was 9,490. During the last months of pregnancy digestion influences the condition of the blood in a third of the cases. This was especially true where either proteid or carbohydrate foods were freely used, but these gave no evidence of insufficient action of the liver. In proportion as the patient had better care the blood cells showed less variation and better development but if the pregnant patient was without proper conditions of living, degenerative forms were seen in the blood cells.

The familiar fact that during pregnancy the excretion of urea is lessened and ammonia coefficient is increased, seems to indicate that the process of producing urea is carried on more extensively than in the non-pregnant. The test of liver function is made by giving the patient, by mouth, organic compounds of ammonia and afterward subjecting the urine to examination. In patients whose livers are healthy, in twenty-four hours following this administration, the urinary salts are quantitatively increased when compared with the urea. If this experiment is to be accurate the diet of the patient must be regulated and the patient must be under observation and care for several days preceding the test. In the writer's experience from 20 to 40 grns. of ammonia citrate were administered and the urine examined and in healthy patients there was no result observed. In others there was a trace of albumin and acid compounds in the urine. In the last months of gestation it was sometimes interesting to give a patient a very rich protein diet and restrict the carbohydrates. Under these circumstances the carbohydrate intake of 120 to 150 Gms. daily, seemed to be sufficient to prevent disturbance in the patient's health.

The feces of the patients in these observations showed no excessive quantity of protein in the matter discharged. These and similar observations go to show that the use of protein food alone in pregnancy, is not a serious factor in producing toxemia.

The **diagnosis of early pregnancy** by recognizing some alteration in the excretions of a pregnant patient has frequently been attempted. Bronnicoff (*Zentralbl. f. Gynäk.*, 1924, 44) reviews the literature of the subject as regards the diagnostic value of glycosuria produced by phloridzin in recognizing early pregnancy. His observations were made in 350 cases of various kinds and in all over 1000 tests were made in 300 women and eight men. Phloridzin was given by intramuscular injection and in another series of 42 men by intravenous injection. By the intramuscular method 1 c.c. of a fresh solution (0.2-100.0) which was 2 Mgms., was given in the morning in the gluteal region. After the injection the patient was told to drink water freely and then the urine was examined for sugar, three times at intervals of half an hour, if necessary it was taken by catheter. Before the injection, a control test was made of the urine to demonstrate the absence of albumin and sugar. In none of these cases was albumin present and the two cases which showed sugar in the urine, were eliminated from the test. In 73.8 per cent of patients in the first two months of pregnancy, the test was positive; in 26.2 per cent the test was negative although the patient was pregnant. In 40 patients who had temporary amenorrhea, 29 gave positive reactions and 11 negative. In 122 patients known to be pregnant, 82 were healthy, 20 tubercular, and 20 anemic. Among the healthy patients 61 gave positive tests and 21 negative tests; in the tubercular 14 were positive and 6 negative. In the anemic 10 were positive and 10 negative.

Cases of incomplete abortion from six weeks to the third month, were also examined, 60 in all, of whom 40 gave a positive and 20 a negative test. In order to control the test 70 cases, 60 of these not pregnant and 10 patients who had passed the menopause, were given this test and with the exception of three, aged 45, 55, and 60, the results were negative. The three patients had prolapse of the uterus and they gave a positive reaction. Twenty-two patients were examined during the menstrual period and 13 gave a positive reaction.

When men were examined 72 per cent gave positive and 14 per cent a negative test. This percentage is the same as that obtained in the examination of women.

These experiments are an illustration of the difficulty in diagnosticating pregnancy because of disturbed metabolism. They should lead to caution in placing too much reliance upon technical results.

*The Treatment of Eclampsia* is always a subject of debate. Zweifel (*Ztschr. f. Geburtsh. u. Gynäk.*, 1923, 39, 1521) reviews the literature and summarizes his clinical experience, and like others he urges the earliest possible detection and treatment of conditions threatening eclampsia. He would first of all introduce fluid into the body of such patients, and if they are unconscious in toxemia, it is injected into the bowel or subcutaneously or with the help of the stomach tube introduced into the stomach. He would wash out the stomach thoroughly and then leave in the stomach a considerable quantity of lemon juice or very dilute vinegar and water. Eight hours after this he would thoroughly irrigate the stomach with normal salt solution and he would also use normal salt solution subcutaneously if not retained in the stomach. He would never use very large quantities lest he might encourage the development of edema.

As regards interfering with pregnancy, expectancy is the better treatment. In observing 317 eclamptic cases, there were 27 who died, four of these had lesions in the lung which indicated that too much fluid had been given, three of these patients got pneumonia because the contents of the stomach entered the bronchial tubes. Of the fatal cases, 15 showed extensive blood disintegration, four died of cerebral apoplexy, and there was one patient who before admission to hospital gave indication of threatened collapse.

In the very beginning of the treatment he has seen excellent results from prompt bleeding; where cerebral apoplexy is threatened, he has obtained the best results by rapid cesarean section and bleeding. In estimating the mortality, if those cases are eliminated which were favorable for treatment in the early stages had they been brought to hospital, the mortality is reduced to 3 per cent; but it must be understood that such a low mortality is not possible unless cases are recognized early and treated efficiently. The difference between indiscriminate and rapid delivery and more conservative methods is shown by fetal mortality of 36 per cent following rapid delivery, and 18.8 per cent where more conservative methods were adopted. If delivery should be practiced, abdominal cesarean section is best. He has seen for some time no cases where decapsulation of the kidneys was indicated, although previously he had seen good results from this operation. He believes it to be important that the stomach and mouth contents, of unconscious patients, do not enter the bronchial tubes.

Stroganoff's method is always interesting in comparison with others. During a recent visit to Edinburgh he stated (*J. Obst. & Gynæc. Brit. Emp.*, 1923, 30, 1), going back to 1913 for statistics, that there were in Europe that year fourteen million confinements with a mortality in 10,000 varying from 3.5 per cent to 5.4 per cent. If the average of four mothers in each 10,000 is taken, 5600 mothers die in England every year of eclampsia and 8400 children. He estimates that 6000 children die yearly in the United States from that cause. In both countries 24,000 mothers and children are lost each year from the toxemia of gestation. New Zealand has apparently the highest mortality, 25 per cent. Stroganoff claims for his method of treatment a maternal mortality ranging from 4.7 to 23.3 per cent. He has several times reported series of cases with a mortality from 5 to 6.6 per cent. He is positive in believing that maternal mortality can be reduced to 1 or 2 per cent by his methods of treatment. He agrees with others that surgical interference is rarely indicated.

As is known, his method consists in removing all irritation, secluding the patient in a dark and quiet room, using chloral hydrate, morphin, and chloroform, and giving milk and salt solution. The patient's treatment is varied somewhat as eclampsia develops before labor, after labor, or during labor. Where the question of weakening the heart's action by chloral is discussed, he believes that from 1 to 1.5 Gms. of chloral hydrate is less depressing to the heart and centers of respiration than the eclamptic convulsion. If patients pass through eclampsia without delivery, the treatment by narcotics is continued, to prevent, if it can readily be done, the appearance of labor; but should labor develop it is assisted in the least violent manner possible. He is often obliged to use stimulation such as digitalis. The mouth and nose must be cleansed frequently and carefully, oxygen administered, pure air, and every effort made to secure successful respiration. He applies heat by hot water bottles around the patient. If three convulsions occur he performs bleeding, taking 400 c.c. of blood. He estimates the amount of blood lost in delivery in normal cases as 800 c.c. and in view of this fact he believes that caution should be exercised in bleeding in eclampsia. The patient is disturbed as little as possible, the stomach and intestines are not molested, the patient is turned from side to side in bed frequently, remaining longer on the right side. If bleeding is practiced, dry cupping is not necessary. He quotes the statistics of Russian hospitals: 78 cases without mortality in one, 152 with four deaths in another, 88 cases without a bad result in another, and taking all the favorable cases, he collected 166 without mortality. Where death did occur, extensive degeneration of the viscera was found. He claims 1.07 per cent maternal mortality with fetal mortality of 5 per cent. The number of convulsions was reduced to 1.3 per cent.

**The Weight of the Parturient Patient During Pregnancy and Labor and the Puerperal State.**—Kemper (*Arch. f. Gynæk.*, Band 121, Heft 2, 1924) finds that three factors influence the weight of parturient women, the initial weight of the woman, the number of pregnancies, age, and the intensity or average rate at which variation in weight develops. When cases are studied in groups and compared, it is found that there is less variation in weight in parturient women during pregnancy and the puerperal state than has been supposed. Even twin pregnancy produces surprisingly little variation.

In discussing the care of pregnant women, the question of the success of so-called antenatal clinics, and the application of their methods to private practice, becomes of definite interest.

At a meeting of the British Medical Association at Bradford in 1924, a discussion occurred on this subject, Fairbarn presiding (*Brit. M. J.*, Aug. 16th, 1924). Willitt, of the City of London Maternity Hospital, stated that their antenatal work began in 1908. They have had no difficulty in examining all primigravidæ and all multiparous patients who had a history of previous complications. Patients are warned at once if any symptom develops, urine is examined each month and the breasts and nipples receive careful attention. When the vomiting of pregnancy is not severe, attention to diet, excretion, and the free use of fruits and the assurance that the patient will improve and recover, are all that is required. Abortion is believed to occur in from 20 to 25 per cent of all pregnancies and there will be no improvement in this percentage until patients place themslves under medical care as soon as pregnancy is known, and also until hemorrhage from the vagina is regarded as a sign of great danger and a symptom to be reported at once.

It is usually possible to detect and treat syphilis in pregnancy satisfactorily. If gonorrhea is discovered the patient is referred for treatment to the department for venereal diseases in a general hospital. In tubercular patients, the management depends upon the social status of the patient and her resources. Cardiac cases, if severe, must enter hospital. In 2145 patients, 204, about 10 per cent, required especial investigation or treatment; 57 had albuminuria but there was no eclampsia although it was feared that many of these cases had chronic nephritis. There was but one case of pyelitis in 104 patients, but wherever there was any symptom of irritation in the region of the kidneys the citrates were freely prescribed. One shoulder presentation and two face presentations were not recognized before labor, the mothers were multiparæ and had normal pelves. Most of these patients were first seen about the twenty-eighth week and breech presentation was not uncommon, in many of these cases the vertex subsequently presented by spontaneous version. It is hopd that the x-ray may give much assistance in recognizing these cases. Where breech presentation is detected, external version is practiced and to dislodge the presenting part, the foot of the patient's bed is raised. Disproportion between mother and child occurred in about one per cent; if the occiput was posterior and deeply engaged, there was no interference. If the head was high up with occiput posterior, manual rotation was tried and late in pregnancy pads and a binder were useful.

The writer's method of pelvimetry was simple and to many satisfactory. He applies the tip of one index finger on the anterior superior spine of the ilium and the tip of the other on the highest point of the crest, between these two points the distance should be not less than 2½ inches which can easily be measured by the eye. The skin is then stretched along the outward edge of the iliac crest and if the patient is lying on her back the normal curve has the convexity downward and backward; if the pelvis is abnormal these conditions are wanting. If there is a suspicion of abnormality the pelvimeter should be used in addition. If one has no pelvimeter the length of the hand from thumb to little finger outstretched, may be used. He finds it important to recognize the landmarks of the fetal head, especially the parietal eminences. If the situation of these landmarks indicate disproportion, if recognized early, they may be an indication for early cesarean section. He believes that the head will mould one half inch without injury. To estimate this the most important guide is the anteroposterior thickness of the pubis. If the pubis is thick and the parietal bone overrides or overhangs the pubis the indication for delivery by section is positive. Examination is made as much as possible by the abdomen, but when difficulty is anticipated, vaginal palpation of the head while pressure is made from above, is of great value. Labor was induced in 24 of 204 patients, in four at full term, in 19 after 36 weeks. There was no maternal mortality, one child was stillborn, and one was delivered by forceps. In 13 cesarean sections the mothers all recovered. In 16 cases going over term, labor was induced without maternal or fetal death. The histories were often obscure among these patients, but in estimating prolonged pregnancy, the rule was made to compute 300 days after the last period. Other signs were also taken into consideration.

Hemorrhage developing during pregnancy was observed in but three cases and such patients must be treated in hospitals only.

These and other similar reports indicate that the principals of prenatal care may be transferred from clinics to private practice with great benefit.

**X-Ray Obstetric Diagnosis Is Always an Interesting and Practical Subject.**—Portes and Blanche (*Gynéc. et Obst.*, 1924, 5) publish a paper giving the results of considerable work in this subject with a large bibliography and three pages of illustrations.

They found this method valuable in diagnosticating pregnancy before signs of fetal life could be recognized, in the diagnosis of multiple pregnancy, pathological pregnancy, mechanical obstacles developing during pregnancy which might influence labor, especially in the diagnosis of disproportion between the head and pelvis. They quote statistics of others who claim to have recognized pregnancy by this method at three and one half months and four months, some at five months and in a series of 24 cases, in one-third of them before the fifth month. The writers studied ten patients with nine negative results and one in which they obtained a positive shadow. In diagnosticating twin pregnancy error can be avoided by the use of the best apparatus in the hands of experienced persons, and if these precautions are taken the method is successful and of great value. In diagnosticating triple pregnancy, there are several cases upon record. Hydrocephalus and monsters can be recognized when the fetus has grown to considerable size. Regarding the question of diagnosticating fetal death in the uterus, there are very few results of practical and proven value in these cases. It is claimed that the recognition of disproportion between the size of the cranium and the size of its contents is positive proof of fetal death. Where maceration occurs, decalcification of the skeleton becomes pronounced and that can be recognized by the x-ray. Tumors complicating pregnancy would suggest examination by this method. In the second half of gestation the x-ray would show the fetal skeleton which would be contrasted with the outline of the tumor.

In ectopic pregnancy the x-ray can render service only after the fetal skeleton is sufficiently advanced to be clearly recognized; so in mechanical complications of gestation, all would depend upon the degree of ossification present in the fetus. So much can be done by this method of diagnosis that it should be kept in mind in all important complications of gestation in which it offers a chance of success.

*An Interesting Case of Primary Chorionepithelioma of the Ovary* is reported by Dougal (*J. Obst. & Gynæc. Brit Emp.*, 1924, 31). The patient was aged 29, in her third pregnancy, and had been in good health until she had a fainting attack and fell, injuring her head, and after being in bed she commenced to have a dark hemorrhagic discharge. For a number of years she had had pain at times in the left lower abdomen. The irregular vaginal bleeding continued about nine months, when menstruation ceased for five and one half months. At times she had vomiting and the abdominal pain had grown worse. On entering the hospital she was thin, slightly jaundiced, normal temperature, pulse about 100. In the abdomen was a very tense tender tumor which felt like a pregnant uterus with concealed hemorrhage. On internal examination there was an elastic swelling in the pelvic cavity which pushed the uterus forward and was continuous with the abdominal tumor. At operation the uterus was extirpated and both appendages removed, and there was a large tumor in the lower abdomen pushing the uterus forward and to the right, with the omentum adhering to the upper surface of the uterus containing vessels of supply. The tumor had grown firmly into the pelvis in the left broad ligament and pushed the rectum over toward the right; the left fallopian tube and ovary could not be seen. The uterus was soft and with the right fallopian tube formed the anterior surface of the tumor. The ovary was large, cystic, and adherent. The tumor was shelled out very carefully and the uterus and tumor removed from before backward and a small dark red nodule was removed from the wall of the rectum. The patient made a good recovery, but returned a week after leaving the hospital with a recurrence of the growth as large as a small orange. This was near the rectum and high up in the pelvis on the left side. On examining the specimen removed, the tumor was a chorionepithelioma of the ovary. There were areas of hemorrhage and masses of Langhans' cells and syncytium and some portions of the tumor showed necrosis and degeneration of the villi.

With his own, the writer collected 11 cases, and also five where the broad ligament was the site of primary chorionepithelioma. Most of these patients were less than 31 years of age, they had had pregnancy usually one or two years before coming under observation. The symptoms were irregular bleeding for a prolonged time and after this cessation of menstruation with constant pain in the abdomen.

Of the 10 cases besides the author's, seven were fatal and three recovered.

**Interference with Pregnancy and Sterilization.**—The effort to make public knowledge concerning birth control is increasing interest in the question of sterilization by surgical means. Freund (*Zentralbl. f. Gynäk.*, 1923, 42) operates by severing the fallopian tube and burying one of the severed ends in the peritoneum and stitching the other end to the abdominal wall. A firm silk ligature is placed around the tube at its junction with the uterus. In 70 cases conception has not followed after the operation and very little shock or disturbance was caused by this procedure.

The effort to secure temporary sterilization is believed by the majority to be impracticable. If the fallopian tube is severed the epithelia degenerate and the natural function of the tube cannot be accomplished. Very often these operations are accompanied by the shortening of the round ligament.

It is possible also to perform this operation, interrupting early pregnancy by the extraperitoneal vaginal cesarean section. Heinsius opens the anterior vaginal wall longitudinally above the cervix, pushes back the peritoneum and without opening it, incises the uterus at the internal os and through the lower segment. Should it be necessary, the peritoneal sac can be opened and, at the termination of the operation, closed by suture.

Sterilization is not effected by this procedure but early pregnancy can be interrupted with comparatively small disturbance to the patient.

Recently the danger of the **cervical attachment of the placenta** has been brought to the attention of the profession by Freund, Humm and other continental obstetricians (*Ztschr. f. Geburtsh. u. Gynäk.*, 1923, Band 85, 581). In Freund's 25 cases, the maternal mortality was 80 per cent. His patients had violent hemorrhage usually following the first cervical and vaginal examination. The behavior of the case is characteristic of advanced cancer of the uterus, and the tissues give a similar sensation to the finger, and the hemorrhage is profuse. It is almost impossible to recognize the cervix, so greatly is it altered. One of the principal causes of bleeding is varicose vessels which develop in these cases. In one patient he could not detach the placenta as the cervix tore during the effort, and he was obliged to extirpate the uterus by abdominal section followed by fatal shock.

In one case Bumm exposed the cervix and ligated the most important vessels and checked the hemorrhage.

These cases were reported before the Berlin Obstetrical Society and the consensus of opinion was that cesarean section in one of the various forms is the only possible means of delivery in this very serious complication.

Under the title *Placenta Accreta,* Polak and Phelan (*Surg., Gynec. & Obst.* Feb., 1924) contribute an illustrated article giving their experience with this complication. They estimate the frequency at 1 in 6000 cases. This condition must be differentiated from simple adhesion of the placenta which is of little importance. Placenta accreta is a definite pathological condition. So completely is the placenta interwoven with the cervix that manual removal is impossible and can only result in hemorrhage, septic infection, or perforation of the uterus. Whenever the expulsion of the placenta is delayed, suspicion should be aroused, and if there is clinical evidence of separation Credé's method should not be tried. Where the placenta is retained without hemorrhage a thorough exploration should be made under anesthesia to decide the method of treatment. If gentle and careful manipulation fail to demonstrate a line of cleavage between the placenta and uterine tissues, hysterectomy or total extirpation of the uterus is indicated.

The writers during the past five years have had eight manual removals of the placenta. Three were partially or completely adherent, but line of separation could be found and the placenta was finally delivered. Four were separate from the uterine wall but were retained by a retraction ring. There was one case in which no line of cleavage could be demonstrated, the placenta was removed piecemeal and not completely, accompanied by such severe hemorrhage that nothing could be done but firmly pack the uterus and give stimulation. While an effort was made to find a donor for transfusion, the patient died, nine hours after admission to hospital. In two other cases the attempt to remove the placenta by manual interference was followed by such hemorrhage that packing was used, but the patients died of septic infection. Both of these cases were multiparæ and previously had had the placenta removed by the introduction of the hand. In a third case narrated the woman was aged 26, married five years without pregnancy. She had had four curettings. When in labor the uterine tumor was very large and a small hard tumor was found just above the pubis in the left lower quadrant. A stillborn seven months fetus was delivered after five hours of labor. The placenta was not expelled and there was no hemorrhage. The uterus contracted intermittently and Credé's method failed to express the placenta. Six hours after delivery, in hospital, under anesthesia and asepsis, the gloved hand found in the lower segment, just above the internal os, a submucous fibroid as large as a grape fruit attached to the anterior left uterine wall, the placenta was above the tumor and no line of separation could be made out. The abdomen was opened and the uterus incised at the right edge of the placenta. An attempt was made to separate the placenta, but this attempt failed. Supravaginal hysterectomy was followed by an uneventful recovery.

**Premature separation of the normally implanted placenta** remains one of the most formidable complications of pregnancy. Scott (*Surg., Gynec. & Obst.*, April, 1924) reports nine cases in the Evanston Hospital, of this complication. He draws attention to the association of toxemia and its probable identification as the cause of the accident. Cases are cited illustrating this contention. One of the cases which he delivered was a primipara aged 30, pregnant seven months, blood-pressure over 200, albumin present in the urine and an increase in the uric acid of the blood. Acute abdominal pain and faintness developed during labor with partial cessation of the pains, which was treated by inserting a dilating bag. In six hours complete dilatation was present and a stillborn child was delivered. Three quarters of the maternal surface of the placenta was occupied by a firm clot. Microscopic section of the placenta showed thickening of some of the walls of the arteries, although the chorionic villi were normal.

The second case was also a primipara with high blood-pressure and edema, delivered by low forceps of a living child. On examination of the placenta, infarcts and a clot were present.

Other illustrated cases are reported. Three cases are studied from the writer's clinic in which the separation came on suddenly and was accompanied by hemorrhage which escaped externally. These patients were treated by prompt delivery, one of them by section, and the recovery of the mothers followed. In two of the three a living child was secured.

From the literature he quotes three cases in which the placenta was delivered, before the child; a stillborn child was spontaneously expelled some time after. In these patients the uterus resembled an ovarian cyst with twisted pedicle; blood had been effused extensively in the uterine wall or under the peritoneum, and one half of the uterus was apparently normal and the other greatly altered. The tendency of the hemorrhage is to separate and draw apart the muscular structure of the uterus forming cysts which are filled with blood. Where successive effusion of blood occurs, round cell infiltration in the neighborhood of these foci has been observed. This process is more pronounced near the fundus and upper part of the uterus and is rarely found in the lower uterine segment. The placental site is most involved and the accident is usually more pronounced on the anteroposterior or lateral aspect of the uterus in accordance with the site of the placenta. The condition is most fully developed and destruction of tissue greatest just beneath the peritoneum; here the uterine wall is literally torn apart by the excessive bleeding.

In nearly all cases the uterine muscle is considerably degenerated and this is most advanced where the bleeding is greatest. This degeneration is not caused by the hemorrhage but is produced by the toxemia which results in the bleeding. In some cases the individual muscle fibers could not be recognized. In the decidua the walls of the vessels are degenerated and there is necrosis of the decidual cells, in the veins or walls of the vessels and where the veins are in direct connection with the effused blood. Thrombosis was present in some cases, infiltration about the vessels in others and there were multiple fissures in the peritoneum sometimes extending into the muscular tissues beneath. This peritoneal lesion was found in 15 per cent of cases. Usually the tear is transverse, sometimes longitudinal, occasionally irregular. These lesions are observed at the fundus on the anterior or posterior wall; as would be expected, they are often at the site of the placental attachment.

In one case, reported by White, among the very earliest, the woman aged 32, in her ninth pregnancy, after giving birth to a dead child, died in about an hour. At autopsy there were peritoneal lesions, extravasations into the broad ligament, and blood was also extravasated into the abdomen. Effusion into the peritoneum was found in 71 per cent. Sometimes this is clear serum and again bright blood.

In 26 of the cases collected, the broad ligaments were involved, the tubes in 11, the ovaries in four, the round ligament in one. Multiform bleeding was the lesion most often found. Extravasation of blood may extend over a very considerable area. The placenta does not seem to be pathological and the only condition found has been slight thickening in the stroma of the ovary. There are the records of 17 autopsies with subcapsular hemorrhage in the liver and acute parenchymatous degeneration. In one case there was hepatic cirrhosis and in one the extreme statement was made that there remained no normal liver tissue. The kidney showed parenchymatous degeneration and there was bleeding in the diaphragm, in two cases; in the pericardium in one, in the meninges one, in the stomach two, and in the adrenals one.

Autopsy on the fetus showed hemorrhage into the viscera. Whether this was caused by asphyxia from placental separation or by toxemia, it is difficult to state.

That placenta prævia and accidental separation can be combined, Scott believes, and supports this belief by the description of two cases in which the mother died and in which the conditions indicated placenta prævia and separation as well. These patients were not seen until the bleeding had become severe. He cites three cases treated obstetrically, as he terms it, in which the mother recovered with the birth of a dead child; delivery was spontaneous. In other patients interference was practiced, and if this was done sufficiently early, the results were favorable.

The writer believes that mild cases of premature separation of the normally implanted placenta are not infrequent. They are toxic and traumatic, the greater portion being toxic. Where the toxemia is mild, small areas of infarction with comparatively slight bleeding develop, which cause the mother but little disturbance, but end in the death of the child. The same toxemia which is seen in eclamptic patients is present in these. If the symptoms are not threatening, the author would use expectant treatment, but if symptoms indicate a condition of severity, delivery by cesarean section is indicated.

**Stimulation of the Uterus.**—*The Method by which the Uterus is Stimulated* has always been of interest to physiologists and especially to obstetricians. Whitehouse and Featherstone (*J. Obst. & Gynæc. Brit. Emp.*, 1923, 4, 565) utilized several abdominal cesarean sections and other operations as well as normal cases, to study the stimulation of the uterus. They added to this experiments upon rabbits and concluded that the nervous mechanism controlling the uterus is local, sympathetic, and lumbosacral and automatic. The local nervous stimulus produces rhythmical contractions of the uterus independently of the other sources of stimulation. This physiological fact is true of other involuntary muscles. The sympathetic nerves increase the action of the circular muscle fibers and inhibit the action of the longitudinal bundles; the nerve centers in the lumbar cord stimulate the longitudinal fibers and inhibit the action of the circular fibers. Centers in the medulla and possibly the cortex, control both automatic and sympathetic stimuli, but these centers can act independently. Reflexes are important factors in normal contractions of the uterus, illustrated by reflexes from the breasts and reflexes set up by stretching or irritating the perineum. To have efficient uterine contractions both automatic and sympathetic nerve systems must be in a condition of health and there must be a balance between them, if there is disability there will be interference with normal labor.

Acting upon these observations the authors conclude that for classic cesarean section lumbar narcosis used alone or combined with general anesthesia, would be advantageous. If this method were employed they would limit the inhibitory stimuli from the lumbar portion of the cord and allow the sympathetic stimulation to produce firm contractions of the circular muscle. This should prevent bleeding. In one of their cases the fetus and five fibroids were removed at full term by operation, with very little hemorrhage. If one can get the circular fibers to contract strongly, the edges of the uterine incision are drawn up which makes the closure of the muscle much easier and more efficient. If there is an indication to increase intra-uterine tension, the use of cocain in the lumbar region should do this and this treatment might be of advantage in premature separation of the normally implanted placenta. In placenta prævia the bleeding might be reduced temporarily by the contraction of the lower segment, but when the placenta was separated the bleeding would increase. In cases of exhaustion during labor, the uterus failing to act, spinal anesthesia should hasten delivery and lessen danger of bleeding. This also should reduce the quantity of blood lost from the placental site. When it is desired to empty the uterus through the vagina in early pregnancy, the writers prefer spinal to general anesthesia. Cases are sometimes seen where the cervix is rigid and a contraction ring develops which greatly retards labor; this is caused by excessive stimulation of the sympathetic system, and in the non-pregnant this may be an important factor in producing dysmenorrhea.

In normal labor spinal anesthesia is not indicated; it will retard the dilatation of the cervix and lessen the expulsive power of the uterine muscle and increase the necessity for the use of forceps.

**Relation of Hemolytic Streptococci to Pregnancy.**—The old question of the relation of hemolytic streptococci to pregnancy and the puerperal period is discussed by Kanter and Pilot (*Surg., Gynec. & Obst.*, Jan., 1924). They quote the literature of the subject and studied 96 patients in the Presbyterian Hospital and Dispensary of Chicago. To obtain the secretion they inoculated swabs, one from the lateral wall of the vagina, the second from the posterior fornix, the third from the os and the cervix. The latter two cultures were taken with sterile speculum and care was taken to avoid the secretions present. They also made studies to determine the possible source of streptococcus infection in puerperal patients, and especially the nasopharynx of the patient and her attendant. They found that the normal vagina rarely contained virulent hemolytic streptococci, nor was there evidence that the presence alone of such streptococci produces puerperal sepsis. Any manipulation or disturbance of the vagina by examination or operation, increases the risk of sepsis. Puerperal hemolytic streptococci infection is considered by most to be exogenous. Drops of secretion from the nasopharynx of the attendant may infect patients and the use of gauze masks is indicated during delivery, and also the exclusion of all persons suffering from sore throat from the delivery room and attendance upon puerperal patients.

That **tuberculous infection of the kidney** can complicate pregnancy is illustrated by Stevens from the San Francisco Clinic (*Surg., Gynec. & Obst.*, Dec., 1924). He reports two cases, one aged 22, and five months pregnant, from whose neck glands had been removed when she was ten years old. The urine showed pus cells. The function of the right kidney was diminished; urine from the left kidney was negative. A guinea pig inoculated from the urine from the right kidney gave a positive reaction to tuberculosis, while inoculation from the left kidney was negative. Consent to operate could not be obtained until after the confinement. The child was delivered by high forceps with a small infected wound on the left side of the neck from which tubercle bacilli were recovered. This wound healed in about three weeks, but later a gland of the same side of the neck suppurated; tubercle bacilli were abundantly present and the child died eight months later from tuberculous meningitis. The mother's kidney was removed and 20 months after the operation she was well.

The second case was aged 30, in the second month, and had a family history of tuberculosis. Tuberculous infection of the bladder was proved by inoculation, and infection of the right kidney. The patient was operated upon followed by marked improvement and abortion two months after the operation. Four months after the operation the remaining kidney was found to be tuberculous.

Stevens reviews 35 reported cases of nephrectomy during pregnancy for conditions other than tuberculosis. The purpose of this review seems to be to determine the possibility of the continuation of pregnancy after this operation. In 26 cases the patient went to term, labor was induced in two, abortion occurred in six, mother and child died in one. In the 17 patients who went to term, the child was normal. In addition to the two reported cases, the writer found 16 cases of nephrectomy in pregnancy for tuberculosis of the kidney; 12 had nephrectomy with recovery of all the mothers; in six a normal child was born at term; abortion occurred in three, and in one of them, two months after the operation; one patient had a dead child at seven months, four and a half months after operation; the death was not due to the operation. The operation was done in all of the months of pregnancy up to and including the sixth. In five pregnant patients having renal tuberculosis who were not operated upon, three became much worse; death occurred in the eighth month in one. In four cases who were not operated on there were two abortions, one child infected at birth subsequently dying, one normal child at term. Obviously all pregnant patients suffering from unilateral renal tuberculosis, should be operated on as soon as the diagnosis can be made. The children born of tuberculous mothers have an average mortality of 58.8 per cent. Following the operation tuberculin should be given, the urine examined often, and the patient kept under observation. If after two or three years the remaining kidney is free from tuberculosis and the woman is in good general health, pregnancy is permissible.

In 261 cases of pregnancy occurring in women from whom one kidney had been removed, there were 250 normal and 15 complicated labors with but two deaths. Should bilateral involvement be present, tuberculin should be given with good hygienic treatment and little will be accomplished for the mother by sacrificing the child.

In the observation of the reviewer a woman from whom one kidney had been removed for tuberculosis, passed successfully through eclampsia and although her child was stillborn she made a good recovery. She was treated by medicinal and obstetric measures only, without operation.

**The management of abortion** is always a subject of prolific discussion. In the *Journal of the American Medical Association* for March 29, 1924, Gordon states the results of his treatment of 1640 cases of whom 961 were minutely studied. These were naturally divided into infected and non-infected, and those were called infected having a temperature above 101° F. by rectum or where there had been interference with the uterus. There were 1528 cases where the abortion was incomplete.

In treatment, on admission the patient was prepared as for labor without interference with the vagina, one vaginal examination only was made. The patient was put to rest in bed and given morphin to quiet suffering, and daily a low enema. Hemorrhage called for active treatment which consisted in removing the products of conception which were in the cervix and partly expelled, by the stick-sponge method. The vagina was thoroughly packed with antiseptic gauze and this manipulation was usually practiced through a speculum. Packing was necessary in 62 per cent of cases of whom 53 were packed once and 10 per cent again. In 38 per cent no packing was required. If the symptoms indicated that abortion was inevitable, 0.5 c.c. of pituitrin was given by hypodermic every three hours for four or more doses. Whether the abortion is complete or not cannot be definitely ascertained without observation extending from five to seven days. The packing introduced is removed in 18 to 24 hours and repeated in 10 per cent of the cases. Septic cases should never receive active treatment. If the patient's temperature is more than 101° F. by rectum, no intrauterine manipulation is permissible. In most septic cases hemorrhage is rare. These patients were placed out of doors if possible in the Fowler's position and feeding was forced, repeated transfusion of small quantities only of blood seemed to help some. Those who were syphilitic received arsphenamin and some had vaccines, sera, foreign protein, and neutroflavin. Careful observation could find no difference in the ultimate results or duration of the illness under any one type of treatment. Conservative treatment properly carried out will fail in less than 4 per cent of cases and mortality and morbidity are in direct ratio with the degree and frequency of uterine invasion. The use of the curet makes septic many originally clean cases. In the 1640 cases, 18 died, 12 of sepsis in whom the curet had been used before admission and three had had abortion induced. One hundred ninety-three patients had sepsis of whom 181 recovered. In the 1640 the curet was used 39 times.

**Formation of Abnormalities in the Placenta.**—The formation of hydatid mole and abnormalities in the placenta have received the attention of Keller (*Gynéc. et Obst.*, 1, 1924). He found in seven cases of hydatid mole, degeneration of the villi caused by alteration in the circulation of the part. In moles the villi are almost completely absent and what are present are the lacunæ which were the original blood channels during the development of the embryo. The origin of these abnormalities in the circulation is at present unknown.

In 116 cases of marginal placentæ, Keller found that an important factor was a fibrous ring in different stages of development at the border of the internal os, where the edge of the placenta came to the edge of the os. In some cases there was necrosis of the villi; in others, of the decidua with hemorrhage. This fibrous ring is sometimes the result of the stagnation of blood in the intervillous spaces at the border of the placenta. This may develop at the sixth or seventh month by the unusual growth of the two placental surfaces. There is then a margin between the two placental surfaces which is outside the chorion. In a small number the placenta is inserted into the uterine cornu; here the chorion is situated at the border of the placental lip which covers the orifice of the tube; that is, fibrin is deposited and the superficial villi increased. The fibrous ring is thus formed outside the chorion. Occasionally one of these placentæ results from the fact that a portion of the decidua reflexa at the placental margin, persists and is not absorbed. A marginal placenta may produce bleeding in pregnancy; this would be followed by partial separation, very rarely by total separation, but often by premature labor. The placenta prematurely separates in these cases not infrequently. In others hemorrhage results because the placenta separates especially where a marginal placenta is at the tubal orifice. Unless the hemorrhage is severe, the condition is often not recognized positively until delivery. The membranes in 116 cases ruptured prematurely; in 17 there was atony of the uterus which is five times more frequent in these than is usually the case.

There is no evidence that this condition interferes with the growth or development of the fetus.

In the *American Journal of Obstetrics* for August 1924, Bagg contributes an illustrated paper showing the result of experiments upon animals with x-ray and other agencies, in the production of malformation. Structural defects in the young are produced by arrested development from disturbances in the circulation. In some impure blood enters the vascular endothelium producing malformation. If such extravasations occur during the critical period in the development of an organ, it may interfere and lead to defect in structure. In experiments, the eyes of animals are readily affected by interference with the animal, because the blood-vessels of the head are often turgid and easily permit the extravasation of blood. In the extremities, club-feet and syndactylism are produced. Sometimes organs like the kidneys are interfered with and may be partially or wholly affected in development. In the unborn, birth injuries by instruments, or pressure by maternal pelvis or partial asphyxia, or increased blood-pressure in the infant during labor, may produce lesions in the head. Small hemorrhages have, however, been found in cases where the child was not subjected to pressure as in those examined in the uterus during cesarean section. From congenital nævi we learn that such blood disturbances may occur before the birth of the child.

The study of the development of abnormal structure adds nothing to our knowledge regarding the cause of club-feet or paralysis and malformation of the lower extremities, but there is distinct evidence of interference in the development of the eyes.

**Leukocytosis and Ectopic Pregnancy.**—That leukocytosis has a relationship to ectopic pregnancy is intimated by Gragert (*Zentralbl. f. Gynäk.*, 1923, 40:17). He finds a normal leukocyte count in ectopic pregnancy where there has been no hemorrhage or inflammation of surrounding tissues. In the absence of these a slightly increased leucocyte count gradually becomes normal. A tubal abortion is usually accompanied by slight hemorrhage which has little effect upon the leukocyte count. This differs very much in different patients as some are greatly irritated by hemorrhage and others are not. After tubal abortion develops, there is a drop in hemoglobin percentage and the number of red cells, the rapidity of this process being in proportion to the severity of the bleeding. Where there is a recent rupture of the tube the blood is markedly altered, the leukocyte count remaining normal. Where the bleeding is gradual but continuous, the leukocyte count is altered. These facts may aid in making a differential diagnosis between inflammatory condition and ruptured ectopic pregnancy. From the leukocyte count and diminution in hemoglobin and red cells, a differential diagnosis cannot be made between ectopic tubal pregnancy and rupture and ovarian tumor with twisted pedicle. If the patient shows normal leukocyte count but a rapid fall in hemoglobin and red cells, it will indicate rupture of the tube and not perforation peritonitis.

Horvat (*Zentralbl. f. Gynäk.*, 1923, 45:1735) reports a case of ruptured tubal gestation with absolute anuria as the extraordinary symptom. After the removal of the ectopic tube, the secretion of urine became normal. The urine tests remained normal and although the patient's recovery was complicated by bronchitis she ultimately did well.

An interesting case of *ectopic pregnancy* was described by Mertens (*Zentralbl. f. Gynäk.*, 1923, 45) in an ovary which showed on removal two cavities filled with blood: in one a corpus luteum filled with blood, in the other placental villi and syncytial cells.

An **ectopic pregnancy in the broad ligament** is reported by Pfeiffer (*Monatschr. f. Geburtsh. Gynaek.*, 1923. Band 65, 85) in a patient aged 28 who had had pain in the lower abdomen and yellowish discharge for one and a half years. Menstruation had been regular without much suffering. About a month after her period she came to the hospital complaining of pain which rendered work impossible. There was no vaginal hemorrhage, the tumor was as large as a fetal head in the abdomen near the uterus. The uterus was enlarged, pushed to the left, the tumor was very sensitive. There was some rise of temperature, and gonorrhea was found in the cervix and urethra. The patient was thought to have pelvic inflammation with pyosalpinx.

With rest in bed the pain became less and temperature normal and after three weeks in hospital, the patient left to return in eight days. The tumor had not become smaller and accordingly the abdomen was opened. There were abundant adhesions between the intestines, omentum, and abdominal wall, and it was necessary to resect a portion of the omentum. The uterus was separated from adhesions and found very little enlarged and the pelvic organs were affected. On the right side the tube seemed normal near the uterus, but then became very much shorter, and terminated apparently at the pelvic wall. The peritoneum on both layers of the broad ligament was intact. The ovary was intact and fairly movable and upon opening the anterior layer of the broad ligament and ligating the vessels, the tumor seemed to be intraligamentary. It was firmly adherent to the internal surface of the ovary. After the tube was tied and separated there was no difficulty in removing the tumor. A corpus luteum could not be found. The left tube was closed as the result of inflammation.

On examining the mass removed, the tube, clot, and villi of the chorion were plainly evident.

The familiar complication of **utero-placental hemorrhage** is reported by Rivière (*Bull. Soc. Obst.*, 1923, 9:543) in two cases. In one lumbar puncture of the child showed bloody cerebrospinal fluid. The child was delivered by forceps, cried feebly on extraction and the placenta was at the fundus and readily detached and delivered with a considerable quantity of blood. The mother recovered without complication, although she had shown some evidence of shock during the labor.

In the second case, a primipara in seventh month, the urine showed a small quantity of albumin and the patient would not permit examination. After a fatiguing day she was taken with violent abdominal pain, hemorrhage, and diarrhea. She became greatly excited, delirious, and very pale, the pulse was regular at 60 and there was moderate external hemorrhage. The uterus was very hard, the cervix firm. No heart sounds could be heard and the lower segment was firmly closed upon the child. Upon admission to the hospital the urine contained a considerable quantity of albumin. At section a reddish fluid was found in the peritoneal cavity, the uterine wall was extremely thin, the placenta was in front and on the right, partly separated by a clot. On the posterior wall of the uterus there were two large ecchymoses, one on each side of the median line. As the uterus contracted and retracted well as the sutures were inserted, it was not removed. The patient's pulse rose to 160 with extreme shock from which she gradually recovered.

That **fever complicating abortion** is of importance is shown by Winters (*Zentralbl. f. Gynäk.*, 1923, 38) by his bacteriological study in the first 12 hours after abortion; in streptococcus infection the mortality was 15.5 per cent, staphylococcus 8 per cent, Bacillus coli communis 3.1 per cent, hemolytic streptococci 20.8 per cent. In general septic infection the mortality was 100 per cent, where pyemia was present 60.6 per cent, diffuse peritonitis 64 per cent. Where there was pelvic peritonitis and pelvic abscess there was no direct mortality, nor was there mortality where the tubes and ovaries were involved or where there was exudate in the pelvis. Under hospital treatment these cases did well. In the attempt to remove the remnants of the ovum, much depended upon the character of the infection present. When hemolytic streptococci were found, the mortality was 30 per cent, where the streptococci were not hemolytic, 16.4 per cent, and 64.5 per cent of cases of abortion emptied the uterus spontaneously. Drugs had little effect in producing this result. In 792 cases without infection, the mortality was 1.1 per cent. The mortality of interference depends largely upon the local conditions present; in general sepsis, 100 per cent mortality results, this is also true in pyemia. When peritonitis is present the mortality following interference is 88 per cent, and where there is inflammation of the tubes and ovaries 25 per cent and there seems to be little difference in the use of the finger and blunt curet, the finger having 3 per cent mortality, the curet 2.6 per cent. Four or five days should pass with comparatively low fever before interference is practiced and bacteriological study should be made of all cases if possible.

**Extra-uterine pregnancy at full term** is reported by Catlin *J. Am. M. Ass.*, Jan. 12, 1924) in a primipara. At the sixth week of gestation she had an attack of pain and faintness. She went almost to term when pain and faintness again occurred and was repeated on the following day and after that pain and fever and she became so ill that food could not be retained and the bowels did not move for two weeks. She was taken to hospital and anesthetized and a pessary placed in the vagina to support the uterus and this was kept in position five weeks. She left the hospital and had another attack of nausea after which she felt better. Fetal movements developed and fetal heart sounds were unusually plain. The child moved excessively on one occasion and then movements ceased entirely. When examined the breasts contained slight secretion, the cervix was soft and the body of the uterus could not be made out. On the left side of the abdomen a bruit could be heard but no fetal sounds. It was thought the uterus contained a dead fetus and it was decided to bring on labor by packing the vagina and cervix with gauze. Four days after this the patient was anesthetized and the cervix dilated and the uterus found to be empty. She was then removed to the hospital where x-ray showed the fetus in a sitting posture with the head at the margin of the ribs and the feet in the left iliac fossa, the back in front, and the shadow of the placenta seemed to be on the left abdominal wall. On section a thin amniotic sac was adherent to the transverse colon and small intestines. It was opened at the edge of the placenta and the fluid carefully removed and the child delivered. It was 55 cm. long and weighed seven and a half pounds and had been dead several weeks. When an effort was made to remove the placenta hemorrhage was so great that it could not be continued. The sac was sewed to the peritoneum and the wound left open and packed with gauze which was changed daily. About 30 days after the operation the entire placenta was removed. The wound was kept packed with gauze and several ounces of 1 per cent dichloramin-T were poured into the cavity daily until it became sterile and the abdomen healed perfectly.

It is believed that the wide open drainage and antiseptic precautions saved the patient. Incision was made along the border of the right rectus muscle and this aided in the rapid closing. The blood vessels at the placental site did not become obliterated until 43 days after the death of the child.

**The Plastic Changes in the Vagina During Pregnancy.**—Runge (*Arch. f. Gynæk.*, Band 122, Heft 3, 1924) has made an elaborate study of this subject to determine the chemical and anatomical changes which go on in the vagina as pregnancy develops. He paid especial attention to the so-called colloid chemistry of the tissue. He distinguishes two stages of the process, one of which develops as pregnancy advances, and the other is accomplished in a comparatively short time during parturition itself.

The first stage, which is gradual, consists in the distention of the elastic tissue with the formation of certain colloid materials which permit a very considerable alteration in the structure of the part. The second stage, which is more acute, the author describes as edema of the vagina developing at the beginning of labor.

The question of **air embolism complicating pregnancy and parturition** has long given rise to discussion. Experimentally it has been reported that air can be injected into the circulation without especial disturbance to the patient; in other cases immediate and the most serious results seem to follow. Hazelhorst (*Arch. f. Gynæk.*, Band 122, Heft 3, 1924) has studied this subject with the aid of the x-ray and illustrates his paper by skiagrams showing the condition of the heart when air has entered the circulation. His researches seem to show that air which enters the right side of the heart, passes with little disturbance to the circulation, into the pulmonary arteries and oftentimes causes no especial result. The air is in bubbles and the effect which it produces depends much upon the size of the bubbles, as the ultimate result is embolism of the larger or smaller terminals of the pulmonary artery. The size of these bubbles of air all depends upon the length of time during which the air remains in the heart and upon the strength of cardiac contractions. The longer the air remains in the chambers of the heart the smaller are the individual bubbles which develop. Where these bubbles of air are greater, the large vessels in the lungs are sooner obstructed and where they are smaller, the obstruction occurs in the vessels of ordinary or smaller size.

When embolism in the vessels of the lungs develops there is a fall in pressure of the circulation at large and a corresponding rise in the pressure in the right heart and the pulmonary vessels. If the heart cannot overcome the disturbance to the circulation, there follows a very essential compression which extends to the left heart and which prevents the distribution of blood to the organs. The heart itself suffers in its nutrition and consequently in the performance of its function. The anemia in the central nervous system which results in this condition increases the general failure of the circulation, and death from venous air embolism results, primarily from emboli in the pulmonary vessels as a result of this insufficient heart action and sudden and intense anemia in the many organs of the body.

So far as practical deductions can be drawn, there seems to be no distinct separation between prophylaxis and therapy. The author warns against conducting obstetric operations with the pelvis of the patient raised. This posture, he believes, causes negative pressure in the veins of the pelvis and favors the entrance of air into the uterus and vagina. Should air have entered, he believes that this position only increases the danger. Where the head of the patient is raised, if air has entered the right side of the heart, the tendency is to limit it to the pulmonary circulation and not to affect the entire system. He recommends for pelvic and obstetric operations, a horizontal position upon the back.

As far as drugs are to be considered, those substances which quickly stimulate the action of the ventricles are useful, such are camphor, caffein, strophanthus, and adrenalin. If possible, puncture of the ventricle should be made as soon as it is seen that air has entered the heart. While this is useful, to be successful from 10 to 20 c.c. of air mixed with blood must be removed to produce a definite result.

The author recognizes the hopelessness of many cases if once a considerable quantity of air has entered the circulation.

**Pregnancy after Nephrectomy.**—Borelius (*Monatschr. f. Geburtsh. u. Gynack.*, Band 67, Heft 6, 1924) cites the cases of six patients who after nephrectomy had one or more pregnancies and were confined under observation in the hospital. Four of these patients had their surgical operations in the hospital, and the histories are available of three cases having six confinements in other hospitals and these were seen and examined by physicians shortly after labor had occurred. The nephrectomies were done for stone in the kidney, tuberculosis of the kidney, and pyelonephrosis. One patient after nephrectomy for stone in the kidney had three normal pregnancies and confinements. One who had a markedly tuberculous kidney removed, had two normal pregnancies and confinements and remained well on recovery from them. One patient had nephrectomy for pyelonephrosis threatening abortion but was finally delivered with forceps. During the puerperal period she had severe pyelitis caused by the colon bacillus. She finally made a good recovery but remained in a highly nervous state. Another patient had a kidney removed for tuberculosis and after that a normal birth complicated by colon bacillus infection, then the removal of an ovarian cyst and after that two normal births, remaining finally in good health. Nine patients had 15 pregnancies after nephrectomy, none had abortion or premature labor, and the pregnancies and labors were normal. It is remarkable how, after nephrectomy, pregnancy proceeds without complications, very few cases had albumin in the urine, none had eclampsia, and all did well. A few of them had pyelitis from which they recovered. In all of these 12 patients, pregnancy occurred some time after the nephrectomy; in three cases nephrectomy was performed during pregnancy and in two of these there was no disturbance in the pregnancy; the third patient had a pyelonephrosis and was threatened with abortion which was checked by morphin and the patient went to term. One patient had symptoms indicating disease of the kidney for 12 years and during this time had two successful pregnancies. During the third pregnancy the condition became so much worse that nephrectomy was performed. A short time after the operation the urine became free from albumin and evidence of tubercular infection disappeared and pregnancy went on without disturbance.

In treating these cases every care was taken to know that the other kidney was healthy, the x-ray was used and the ureters were catheterized to make sure of this important point. In one case nephrectomy was performed although the urine from the other kidney was cloudy with trace of albumin, leukocytes and a few tubercle bacilli; the result, however, was good.

The weight of the children born after nephrectomy varied from 2850 to 3740 Gms. which is the usual weight. In most cases the right kidney was the one affected and removed.

The author quotes the literature of the subject which shows that the experience of other operators has been practically identical with his own. Where one kidney has been removed for tuberculosis and the second becomes involved, pregnancy usually causes so rapid and severe increase in the tubercular process that fatal result soon develops. Most authorities believe that pregnancy influences tuberculosis of the kidney very unfavorably, tuberculosis of the bladder often develops and the ureters may become distended by retention of septic material and the tendency is for the disease to progress during pregnancy and the puerperal state. The question whether marriage should be forbidden in women in whom one kidney has been removed, may be answered in the negative provided the remaining kidney is healthy and the general health of the patient is good and from one to two years should have elapsed after the nephrectomy.

**Changes in the Ovaries Produced by a Blighted Ovum.**—Küstner (*Monatschr. f. Geburtsh. u. Gynaek.*, Band 67, Heft 6, 1924) cites the case of a woman aged 28 who had two spontaneous labors and no abortions and no severe illness. She believed herself to be pregnant and pregnancy was complicated by the spontaneous expulsion of a blighted ovum. Hemorrhage continued and became severe. The uterus was curetted and the diagnosis made of chorionepithelioma. When the patient was admitted to the hospital examination showed a tumor on the left side of the uterus about as large as a hen's egg which seemed to be connected with the uterus by a thin pedicle. The right ovary was somewhat large. There was a bloody secretion but no definite hemorrhage. Material removed for examination showed mucous membrane of the uterus with chorionic cells and characteristic appearance of malignant chorionepithelioma. The uterus and both tubes and ovaries were removed by abdominal section. Examination showed the characteristic lesions in the uterus and also in both ovaries. In the left side was a small mass as large as a cherry which proved to be malignant. On examination syncytial tissue was found throughout all material removed.

The second case was that of a primipara aged 24 with a similar history and with similar pathological findings at operation. The interesting feature is that a very considerable time elapsed between the expulsion of the blighted ovum and the extirpation of the uterus by operation. The changes in the ovaries were characteristic and fairly well developed.

In the third case the changes in the ovaries did not show increase in lutein cells but otherwise the condition was the same.

In a fourth patient, aged 47, the operation consisted in removing the uterus and left tube and ovary allowing the right to remain. The characteristic lesions were found on examination. In a fifth case the findings were essentially those of the first.

In all of these patients there had been a blighted ovum expelled; lutein cells and corpus luteum cysts were present in cases where a blighted ovum was expelled, and also where chorionepithelioma had developed. Apparently changes in the ovaries begin at the same time that the blighting of the ovum takes place. Ordinarily when a blighted ovum is removed, changes in the ovary gradually disappear but in the cases mentioned and undoubtedly in others, the process goes on to the formation of a malignant growth.

**The Notification of Puerperal Sepsis.**—This subject has for a long time occupied the attention of the British obstetrical profession (*Brit. M. J.*, Nov. 5, 1924). A recent discussion was conducted by several societies and the question arose as to whether the regulation proposed could be carried out. This regulation provides that when there is a rigor or temperature of 102° F. or higher for 24 hours, during the first ten days after confinement or abortion, that the case must be reported. The term puerperal fever is to be dropped and in its place puerperal sepsis is to be used.

In discussion it was shown that in some parts of the country the number of deaths from puerperal fever is larger than the number of cases actually reported. Some in discussion urge that septic cases be reported and thus that the patient be brought promptly under efficient treatment. It was thought by some that the term puerperal fever must be retained because it is understood by non-professional persons. A better supervision of obstetric practice is greatly desired. Eden believes that the notification of puerperal fever is not satisfactory. Fothergill estimated that not 4 per cent of the cases are reported; many of these undoubtedly occur after criminal abortion. The difficulties of the general practitioner were emphasized because frequently cases which he treats are found to be under practically the control of midwives who do not practice aseptic precautions.

On the whole it was thought that notification of the complications of pregnancy and labor and the puerperal state was greatly to be desired and if possible, should be enforced.

**Prognosis of Pyelitis Complicating Pregnancy.**—Naujoks (*Zentralbl.*

*f. Gynäk.*, 1924, 47) contributed a paper upon this subject from observations made in Winter's Clinic at Königsburg. His material comprised about 100 cases occurring during 20 years in the hospital of the Clinic. In these patients 21 had been thoroughly examined after their recovery from the disease, functional tests had been made of the activity of the kidneys and every effort taken to secure accurate observation. Of the 21 there were 8 who were subjectively and objectively well. They felt well, examination of the urine showed no abnormality, and the urine taken from the bladder and from the ureters also was sterile. Four patients complained of pain in the back and in the sides and other vague sensations although the urine was free from bacteria, nor was there evidence of disease in the bladder or ureters. In three of the cases a pelvic condition was found to account for the pain and the fourth diffused from dysmenorrhea. There was no evidence that these patients had not recovered from the pyelitis and their complaints indicate how difficult it is to always arrive at a correct diagnosis in these cases.

Of the 21 then, 12 could be taken as in every way well. Of these 12, 10 had had the colon bacillus, one the proteus, and in one the exact nature of the infecting germ was uncertain. There were 9 patients examined after recovery of whom 8 had not made a good recovery. In 7 the colon bacillus was found in the pelvis of the kidney, in one, 13 years after the original illness, there was a mixed infection of the pelvis of the kidney and symptoms of kidney stone. There was usually chronic cystitis in these cases. One patient, 12 years after she had passed through a pregnancy and pyelitis, had a spontaneous premature labor and in a subsequent pregnancy had pernicious nausea which required interruption of pregnancy at four months and was followed by extensive purulent inflammation which caused death. There were 37 cases where pyelitis had been observed from two to thirty years previously and of these one had had a return, 23 remained in good health, 8 had not recovered from the original attack and 5 could not be traced.

It is customary in this clinic to treat pyelitis during pregnancy in a very conservative manner. In these cases catheterization of the ureter was performed 14 times, in but one only was the pelvis of the kidney irrigated, and in only one case was therapeutic abortion practiced. Reliance was placed upon rest, hygiene, warm applications, and those substances which seemed to disinfect the urine and this, the author believes, is the safer form of treatment.

**Contracted Pelvis.**—In the *British Medical Journal* for February 2, 9, and 16, 1924, are published three lectures by Fitzgibbon, Master of the Rotunda Hospital, on this subject. He states that the obstetrician should consider a pelvis contracted when its size or contour interferes with spontaneous delivery. Lesser degrees of contraction are especially dangerous because they do not occur in deformed women and often do not attract attention. Apparently small women frequently have successful labors so that it is not the actual stature of the patient which is important.

He states that a normal pelvis has an anteroposterior diameter of 4 1/5 inches or 10.5 cm. and a transverse diameter of 5¼ inches or 13 cm. at the brim. The cavity is practically circular, varying from 4¼ to 5 inches in diameter. When the outlet is dilated it is practically circular with the average diameter of 4½ inches. The average normal infant weighs from 7 to 7¼ pounds and both diameters which engage in the pelvis in spontaneous labor measure 3¾ inches. It is important to remember that the size of the fetal head can be reduced by pressure. When one studies the ratio of the fetal head to the pelvis it is found that spontaneous delivery is possible more often than has been supposed. No general classification can be made which is practical but each case must be studied and treated on its merits on careful observation. While the degree of contraction may greatly alter the prognosis it very often does not exclude delivery through the pelvis.

The author is accustomed to study cases during actual labor where there is no great pelvic contraction or disproportion and if this be done accurately and early, from 70 to 80 per cent of cases of contracted pelvis terminate with no more difficulty than normal cases. Those requiring obstetric surgery can be taken to hospital and receive proper treatment before complications develop. If a patient with contracted pelvis can deliver herself, labor does her no harm, and injuries arise from prolonged or ineffectual labor which develops gradually.

He divides contracted pelvis into (1) symmetrically contracted, (2) small round or transversely contracted, (3) generally contracted flat pelvis, and (4) small flat pelvis. He draws attention to contraction of the anteroposterior diameter as the most important element influencing the prognosis for delivery. The transverse diameters are rarely reduced to any extent. In one year the author met 190 cases of contraction of the pelvis. These did not include those having an external conjugate of more than 18 cm. except among the round pelves and two cases with marked difficulty in flat pelvis. The average external measurements of these 190 were 23.25 cm. between the spines, 25.85 cm. between the crests, external conjugate 17.78 cm. The average weight of the infants was 7 pounds 3 ounces. In 99 consecutive cases treated by cesarean section for contracted pelvis in another hospital, the measurements were 9.2 inches between the spines, 10 inches between the crests, external conjugate 7.2 inches, and the average weight of the children 6 pounds 14½ ounces.

Symmetrically contracted pelvis the author considers usually as hereditary. Among these patients the proportion of low forceps application was not greater than the average. In one case, because progress lingered, section was done when it was found that the head had passed the brim so completely that it was necessary to use forceps to bring it up again. Among these patients 14.4 per cent required interference.

Sixty-nine cases of transversely contracted or small round pelves were seen; the anteroposterior diameter was from 20 cm. to 17 cm. These were among the most dangerous cases so far as the transverse diameter was concerned and there was marked difficulty in delivery. In 14 vertex presentations among these cases there was marked difficulty at the brim where the head lodged. In two cases where the head passed the brim, the child was stillborn. Forceps were used more frequently than normally and the head was often excessively moulded; 29 per cent of these cases were difficult.

There were 70 cases of generally contracted flat pelvis, the anteroposterior diameter not greater than 18 cm., and this produced no effect on delivery. One large child was delivered by low forceps followed by death from intracranial bleeding. Forceps delivery was not more frequent than the average. Two patients were delivered by section, one for a second time, although the children were about average size; one in her third labor had version. In a primipara the cord prolapsed with very slight dilatation of the cervix, the fetus died and the patient was delivered by craniotomy.

In 18 cases of small flat pelves the external conjugate was as low as 15½ cm. There was difficulty in labor in 3 cases, 18.75 per cent, and forceps were used more often than the average. Thirty-three rachitic cases were studied in which the iliac crests were involved and gave evidence of the disease; rachitis, however, does not produce any one definite type of pelvic contraction, nor is it a very serious complication in labor and only five out of 33 patients had any difficulty.

In the whole series of 190 contracted pelves, 20 per cent had difficulty in labor. Cesarean section was performed ten times, pubiotomy eight, forceps delivery seven, perforation after prolapse of the cord in one. Eight children were stillborn or died soon after delivery, of whom one was delivered by section, four by pubiotomy, and two by version and one perforated; as the section was done early in labor there was no evident cause for the death of the child. Forceps were used in 12.1 per cent and there was more moulding of the head than normal in these cases. In all cases in the hospital during this time the forceps were used in 7.3 per cent and in primiparæ in 16.66 per cent. This would indicate that forceps need not be used more often than the average in contracted pelves.

The writer places little importance upon contraction at the outlet of the pelvis. In his experience if the brim will allow the head to pass, there will be no greater difficulty at the outlet. He has never had difficulty in extracting the head after it has reached the outlet. He believes that cases reported of deformity of the outlet are really those of disproportion at the brim and that this is not noticed until the head lodges in the pelvis. The difficulty in delivery arises from disproportion during the passage of the head to the outlet and consequent interference with mechanism. He does not measure the outlet but in the reports of other hospitals in 261 cases, 65 were reported as contracted at the outlet, of whom 41 ended in spontaneous delivery, 19 were terminated with forceps, one by section, and 4 not accounted for. He does not believe that one can estimate accurately the size of the fetal head before the test of labor. Women with contracted pelves tend to produce small children but not always small enough to balance the contraction of the pelvis. The principal indication of disproportion is the head high and movable above the pelvis, the soft tissues keep the head high more often than the pelvis does.

Fitzgibbon divides contracted pelves into minor, medium, and major groups. In the minor the true conjugate is larger than 9 cm. and the prognosis for pelvic delivery is good. In the medium the anteroposterior diameter is reduced to 9 cm. but not less than 8, and transverse not less than 10.75 cm. If the bitemporal diameter of the head can be substituted for the biparietal in these cases, spontaneous labor is possible and this depends upon the transverse diameter of the pelvis. He had 157 such cases and 14.6 per cent had very marked difficulty in labor. When the true conjugate is reduced to 8 cm., pelvic contraction becomes the major degree and a normal transverse diameter does not help. Of these he had 6 cases, of which 34.6 per cent had difficult labors.

Diagnosis should be made in prenatal clinics before labor and the conjugate and two transverse measurements, he believes, are most important. If the conjugate is less than 19 cm. the cavity of the pelvis is lessened. He used Skutsch's pelvimeter for internal pelvimetry. Radiography be believes impracticable. The fetal head and the pregnant condition obstruct the pelvis and he thinks that during labor patients cannot be transported to hospitals to obtain an x-ray picture of the pelvis and an expert is not always available to read the plates after they have been obtained. In emergency one often can not get an x-ray picture.

Contracted pelvis does not influence pregnancy until the thirty-sixth week when descent should occur. The end of the thirty-sixth week is the best time to examine a case of contracted pelvis; complete examination under anesthesia may be indicated and about 70 per cent of cases will show good proportion and can go on safely to term. Cases of contracted pelvis should come into hospital at a calculated date for observation and treatment. Palpation and internal measurements are most valuable in studying these cases. If the promontory of the sacrum can be reached by vaginal examination, the internal conjugate is not more than 9 cm. The lateral edges of the brim should also be palpated and the relation of the head to the pelvic brim is most important. Where the head lodges against the top of the pubis the condition may be a grave one. If the head enters the brim the pregnancy may go on 10 to 14 days longer, but if the head impinges against the thumb of the examiner the head usually will not enter the pelvis and the pregnancy should be terminated. If induction of labor is to be performed, it must be done promptly so soon as the disproportion is recognized.

In the first stage of labor contracted pelvis does not seriously interfere with the normal presentation; if the membranes rupture prematurely, then abnormality may develop. During the second stage of labor the influence of pelvic contraction is greatest, the cervix usually draws up leaving the head against the pelvic brim. In the second stage, moulding is not excessive if the cervix continues to dilate. If this does not occur, the lower segment stretches and presses constantly upon the head and there is considerable moulding. Well marked moulding is evidence of disproportion.

As to the mechanism of labor in contracted pelvis: where the transverse diameter of the brim is lessened the head may be forced through with the posterior fontanelle last and with excessive flexion. In small flat pelves the head moves laterally and accommodates itself to the brim; there is not much flexion until after the brim is passed and the head is flattened transversely; impaction results when the proportions between the head and pelvic brim are such that the head can engage but cannot be reduced by pressure sufficiently to pass. Contracted pelvis often calls for unusual uterine force and this may be followed by inertia or overdistention with rupture.

In treatment Fitzgibbon recognizes three methods: (1) spontaneous delivery which includes the use of forceps after the obstruction is passed if excessive moulding is not present; (2) the induction of labor; and (3) cesarean section. During pregnancy the induction of labor is the only treatment to be considered. At term the choice lies between spontaneous labor, or delivery by section. In inducing labor any time four weeks before full term may be selected. It is rarely necessary to induce labor as early as the end of the thirty-sixth week; more cases are taken at the end of the thirty-eighth week and induction of labor is indicated in 25 per cent of all pelvic contractions. His method is to introduce a small rubber tube, under careful aseptic precautions. If there is marked obstruction, cesarean section is usually indicated, although he believes that over 70 per cent of cases of pelvic contraction will deliver themselves spontaneously, under good care and observation. If the membranes bulge in a large bag into the vagina with the cervix partly dilated, section is usually required. Examination under anesthesia is very valuable. If the head has not passed the brim and the membranes have ruptured, vaginal examination is made within a half hour. If the cervix is fully or nearly dilated, and the head engaged with slight overlapping, the head will come down in a reasonable time and may be delivered safely with forceps. Labor may still go on if the cervix is only partly dilated if the head has entered the brim as a vertex and the cervix is closely fitted around the head. If the membranes have ruptured and the cervix is not applied to the head but remains as a vaginal portion, section is indicated in not less than six hours. A second vaginal examination should be made in all cases not delivered within four hours after the rupture of the membranes. Where the anterior lip is thickened and greatly lengthened, the head is greatly moulded, the occiput may be posterior and the parietal bone may be presenting, spontaneous labor cannot be expected and the use of forceps may cause the death of the fetus in 50 per cent of the cases. In proper cases pubiotomy may be performed but section is safest. These cases are serious because the forceps is often applied and failure of this attempt greatly militates against the success of operation.

Where a considerable portion of the vaginal part of the cervix has reformed, with partial closure of the internal os, the head high above the pelvic brim, section is indicated. The writer believes that cases are no less suitable for section four hours after rupture of the membranes than at the beginning of labor.

High forceps in contracted pelvis do more harm than good, in some cases pubiotomy makes the use of forceps successful. These cases should never be allowed to go to the point of great distress for the mother and forceps should be used on maternal indications. The forceps should complete delivery where the natural forces have failed to do so but have overcome the obstruction, and before the vitality of the patient is reduced by the useless prolongation of labor. Version, he believes, has no place in the treatment of contracted pelvis. Pubiotomy is easy to perform, safe for the mother, and saves the child. In the last four years the author has performed the operation 18 times, with the delivery of 13 living infants. Two mothers, previously infected, died; the child of one of these survived. He would never, however, with considerable disproportion and difficulty, allow labor to go on with the definite decision to perform pubiotomy; in all doubtful cases he would perform section. Craniotomy is usually proof of failure in treatment.

In a year the writer had 110 spontaneous normal deliveries with the death of three infants; one low forceps with the death of two infants; five low forceps with marked moulding, and no mortality; two high forceps with no mortality; four pubiotomies with no mortality; fifteen cesarean sections with two infant mortalities; eight induced labors with death of one child; five induced labors terminated by low forceps, no mortality; two craniotomies; two prolapse of the cord terminated by forceps; three easy breech labors without accident; two face presentations converted into vertex; four twin cases without mortality; eight premature children of whom five died; and two cases of macerated children; 184 deliveries with fetal mortality of 19.

Pelvic measurements averaged 7.12 inches for the external conjugate, the maximum being 7.6 and the minimum 6.6. The distance between the crests averaged 10.2, the maximum being 11.6 inches, the minimum 8.2.

# DISEASES OF THE VULVA

FREDERICK JOSEPH TAUSSIG, M.D.

## APPENDIX

**Anatomical Variations of Bartholin's Gland.**—There exists considerable variation in the location and size of the glandular structures about the vulva. These consist primarily of four types of glands: (1) The sebaceous glands situated in the mons veneris, the labia majora and minora and the genitocrural fold, that secrete a white, claylike, ordorous material; (2) sweat glands, found in about the same area, giving to the vulva its glistening appearance; (3) mucous glands situated around the clitoris, to either side of the urethra (corresponding to the prostate gland in the male), and around the insertion of the hymen; many of them having a duct that can be probed; and (4) the large vestibular glands, so-called Bartholin's glands. Melnikoff [1] has recently made a detailed study of the variations in conformation and location of Bartholin's glands. They are first visible in sections of the embryo at the tenth or eleventh week and develop slowly until puberty when they become definitely palpable structures about 1 cm. in diameter. Even in the same individual they may vary considerably in size. In general the greatest diameter is 1.5 to 2 cm. It is often impossible to determine by the size alone the presence of an infection. The gland itself in over half the cases lies somewhat below the line of the posterior commissure. In the remaining 40 per cent it lies to the side of the vaginal outlet. On the other hand the opening of the duct is situated somewhat higher, and in cases of perineal laceration there may be a dislocation of the meatus of the gland so that it is nearer the urethra than the perineal fold. Of special interest are the reduplications of this duct, occasionally leading to a double meatus on one or both sides.

**Treatment of Bartholinitis.**—The unsatisfactory results in the treatment of infections of Bartholin's gland, especially those due to gonorrhea, has led to several new therapeutic suggestions. Huebner [2] injects the patient's own blood in the periphery of the gland and in all 10 cases reported obtained a complete cure of the infection. In three instances the injections were repeated. Sieber [3] had a surprisingly satisfactory result with x-ray in an acute gonorrheal infection of this gland.

He employed a 3 mm. aluminum filter, a field 6x8 cm. in size and 80 per cent H.E.D. as a dose. This treatment was repeated on four successive days. Already on the third day gonococci were absent in the secretions. One month later after an injection of 0.5 Gm. arthigon as an excitant, a few gonococci could again be found in the duct of the gland. Now a final treatment with 0.5 mm. zinc as a filter, 1 H.E.D., was given with permanent result. He suggests a further trial of this therapeutic measure.

**Vulvovaginitis in Children.**—Kahn [4] on the basis of 207 cases distinguishes two forms, one a simple catarrhal form, due to chemical, thermic, or mechanical irritation and the other, a bacterial form. In the bacterial group we must differentiate those due to gonorrhea from those due to other bacteria. The latter he terms "pseudogonococcic vulvovaginitis." In the gonorrheal form he finds an autogenous vaccine of value. If this is not available, a polyvalent diplococcus vaccine is recommended. Other treatment consists of salves or irrigations with silver albuminate preparations and, above all, increasing the resistance by strengthening the body.

**Anatomy and Physiology of the Clitoris.**—Heyn [5] gives the measurements of the clitoris as ranging between 0.5 to 5.0 cm. in length, 2 to 15 mm. in thickness and 5 to 7.5 mm. in transverse diameter. Among older writers the statement is often found that in tropical countries and especially among the black races the clitoris is larger than among the white. There is no real evidence supporting this. This impression probably originated from the fact that the labia majora are smaller in the blacks, thus leading to increased prominence of the labia minora and clitoris but without actual increase in size. There is also no evidence showing that the increased size of the clitoris is the result of increased sexual activity. Out of 1000 women he found a large clitoris (4 cm. or more) in 1.6 per cent only, whereas 33.7 per cent of these women evinced a greater amount of sexual activity. It would seem that the size is more the result of congenital formation than hypertrophy. Where a large clitoris is present, however, there is usually excessive sexual irritability.

That the clitoris is an essential factor in the production of the orgasm in women and so is a factor also in sterility, has been definitely disproved. Out of 529 women the vagina was found to be the important factor in orgasm in 362 or 68.4 per cent, whereas the clitoris was the sensitive spot in only 159 or 30 per cent of these cases. Of the latter group only 23.2 per cent reached the state of orgasm constantly, whereas in the group with vaginal sensibility the percentage of regular orgasm was 40 per cent. It is therefore untrue that a small clitoris is in any degree a factor in sterility or lack of sexual excitement.

**Variations in the Morphology of the External Genitals.**—While in general there is a wide range in the normal aspect of the external genitals slight abnormalities may serve as a valuable index of the sexual development of the patient. The vulva is one of the most important of the secondary sex characters. It represents fairly accurate a mirror of ovarian function. The extent and distribution of hair-growth, according to Labhardt,[6] indicate often a more masculine type with growth over the entire thighs, associated ofttimes with scanty menstruation. Mention has already been made of variations in the size of Bartholin's gland and the clitoris. The perineum also varies greatly both as to its height and as to the presence or absence of a special frenulum. Occasionally an ovarian tumor is associated with a hyperdevelopment of the vulva and this same condition has also been noted in tumors of other ductless glands as in Babcock's case of hypernephroma.

**Unusual Tumors of the Labia.**—Ferguson [7] describes a pendulous tumor of the left labium majus, which developed after a fall and was at first diagnosed as an unusual variety of levator hernia. An exploratory laparotomy showed no connection with the upper pelvic organs and a short time later the tumor was itself removed. It was found to be elongated and in close relationship to the rectum extending forward under the symphysis. The tumor mass measured over 2 feet in length after removal and microscopic examination showed a telangiectatic fibromyoma with hyaline degeneration and edema. The patient made a good recovery from the operation.

Kardschieff [8] describes a somewhat similar tumor which he calls a fibroteleangioma of the labium majus. He believes the point of origin in his case to have been the corpora cavernosa of the labia majora.

Cystic tumors of the labia minora according to Mondor and Huet,[9] usually contain a viscid, colorless fluid. Cholesterin crystals are often found. These authors favor the theory of an origin from wolffian remnants. Thirty-eight cases in literature are reviewed. Bonaretti [10] has also recently described a double cyst of the labia minora, whose origin he attributes to remnants of the Müllerian ducts. Both cysts were the size of a hazelnut. In view of the absence of any embryological relation between the vulva and the wolffian or Müllerian ducts it seems impossible that they have any real etiologic significance. What has been said at the beginning of this chapter about glands normally found about the labia and vestibulum offers a more plausible explanation of the point of origin of these cysts.

**Treatment of Pruritus Vulvae.**—Results of x-ray therapy in pruritus of the vulva vary considerably. Siegfried Meyer [11] finds that with suitable dosage 60 per cent out of 46 cases were fully cured, and all were partly relieved. In case of recurrence of the pruritus a second course of x-ray treatment will usually give the desired result. On the other hand, Werner [12] failed to get any improvement in half of the 51 cases of his series. In view of the association of the pruritus with ovarian disturbances he is inclined to attribute the favorable results rather to distant action on the ovaries than to a local effect on the vulval nerve endings. He therefore favors direct raying of the ovaries together with the administration of ovarian extract. In this connection it is of interest to observe that good results have been obtained by Langhans [13] with psychotherapy in the form of hypnosis in cases of pruritus associated with kraurosis.

**Relation of Vulval Diseases to Fertility, Pregnancy and Labor.**—In the section on diseases of the vulva of Halban-Veit's handbook on *Biologie und Pathologie des Weibes,* Volume III, A. Labhardt gives a good review of the relation of fertility and childbirth to these diseases.

*Fertility* can be hindered by conditions producing a mechanical obstruction such as an imperforate or rigid hymen. At times this structure is so thick and fleshy that it requires incision and even excision to permit of sexual relations. The fact that occasionally pregnancy will occur with an intact hymen is however evidence that it is not always necessary for the immission of semen to take place within the vagina. That large tumors of the labia or extensive cases of chronic hypertrophies of the vulva will prevent sexual relations is self-evident. A not infrequent hindrance follows operations for perineal repair that leave a small vaginal opening with a firm unyielding scar-tissue ring at the introitus. Occasionally the sclerosis following kraurosis of the vulva or the scars associated with extensive vulval ulcerations will prevent coitus and so produce sterility. In addition to these mechanical obstructions, we have also to consider certain inflammatory conditions that make sexual relations impossible and so lead to sterility. These inflammations are usually chronic and associated with severe pain when they are touched. The most common of these conditions are caruncles of the urethra, and the condition known as vaginismus, or vaginal spasm, hindering coitus, often results.

*Pregnancy* produces many changes about the vulva owing to the obstruction of the venous and lymphatic return. Varicose veins may develop of such size as to require a compression bandage for their relief.

Edema is at times present, especially in the presence of heart or kidney complications. Condyloma acuminata are prone to appear in the presence of an acute gonorrhea and develop to considerable size by the conclusion of the pregnancy. In the puerperium these condylomata usually disappear spontaneously. Mycotic vulvitis is not rare during pregnancy associated with a similar infection of the vagina. Herpes of the vulva has also been observed. In the presence of a furunculosis during pregnancy it is very important to eliminate the infection as rapidily as possible since it may prove a complicating factor at the time of labor in predisposing to puerperal infection. Vulval tumors, such as carcinoma or sarcoma, are rarely found in women during the child-bearing years.

*Labor* is only rarely complicated by diseases of the vulva. Large vulval tumors, especially if associated with sclerosis or scars about the introitus, may prove a hindrance. Yet in the case of the large pendulous tumor described in my monograph, page 111, there was no difficulty in either of the two deliveries occurring after its development. Furunculosis, vulvitis, and Bartholin abscess are more serious complications owing to the danger of infection. Labhardt tells of two patients who lost their lives from puerperal sepsis resulting from furunculosis of the vulva. Hence he advises applications of tincture of iodin to the vulva before and after delivery in such cases. Varicosities of the vulva require special care to prevent rupture of a large vein during labor with resulting hematoma of the vulva.

## LITERATURE


1. Melnikoff. Ztschr. f. Anat. u. Entwickl.-geschichte, 1923. 62: 493-520.
2. Huebner. Deutsche med. Wchnschr., 1924. No. 1.
3. Sieber. Zentrlbl. f. Gynäk., 1924. 48: 2126-2130.
4. Kahn. Arch. f. Gynæk., 1924. 121: 335.
5. Heyn. Zentralbl. f. Gynäk., 1924. 48: 40-41.
6. Labhardt. In Halban-Seitz, Biologie und Pathologie des Weibes, III, 1195-1199. (See also literature on Diseases of Vulva, 1254-1260.)
7. Ferguson. Edinb. M. J., 1924. 31: 149-157.
8. Kardschieff. Inaug.-Diss., München, 1922. Rev. in Zentralbl. f. Gynäk., 1924. 48:2103.
9. Mondor and Huet. Gynéc. et obst., 1923. 7: 26.
10. Bonaretti. Arch. di ostet. milan., 1923. 17: 315.

11. S. Meyer. Inaug.-Diss., Breslau, 1923. Rev. in Zentralbl. f. Gynäk., 1924. 48:983.
12. P. Werner.. Wien. klin. Wchnschr., 1924. 37, No. 13.
13. Langhans. Inaug.-Diss., Heidelberg, 1922. Rev. in Zentralbl. f. Gynäk., 1924. 48: 516.

# SURGERY OF THE FEMALE PELVIS

CAREY CULBERTSON, M.D.

## APPENDIX

### POSTOPERATIVE MANAGEMENT AND COMPLICATIONS

The management of convalescence following surgical operations commences with the return of the patient to her room where she at once comes under the care of a specially detailed nurse. The room has been freshly aired and is at a temperature of 68° or 70° F. The bed is warmed by an electric pad or hot water bottles in flannel bags, the light is subdued and only those necessarily in attendance are admitted to the room. In hospital practice it is desirable that there be maintained, in a quiet wing of the building, a small recovery ward to which patients occupying ward beds are brought for the ensuing two or three days.

During the time that the patient is unconscious and relaxation complete her head is turned to the side, without a pillow beneath, and the lower jaw is supported until there is no longer danger of the tongue falling back over the flaccid glottis. Under the more advanced methods of anesthesia, however, such prolonged relaxation seldom obtains, so that by the time the patient is back in her room consciousness is either restored or is returning. Where such is not the case, oxygen gas may be administered and the foot of the bed elevated, thus assisting in overcoming shock or even a tendency toward shock.

Even when drainage has been employed, lowering of the head is a wise precaution for a few hours following operation, and is always indicated when this has been an unusually serious one, unduly prolonged, exceptionally traumatic, or attended by more than the ordinary loss of blood. Only rarely is it necessary to place the patient in the Fowler position immediately.

As a rule, for the first two or three days, the patient will be most comfortable on her back, her head on a pillow. The greatest relief from suffering accompanies the most complete rest, and turning her from side to side only increases pain. Moderate flexion of the legs by placing a pillow beneath the knees affords a measure of relief at times. Only in the exceptional cases demanding abdominal drainage is the lateral position of advantage and, when this is indicated, the lateroprone attitude is best.

The reaction to major operations is so severe that the patient is usually quiet, commotion being more frequent after minor or plastic procedures. Restraint, while seldom required, may become necessary in the case of the neurotic or hysterical person who is noisy and may even attempt to escape from bed. In case of the patient subject to some definite mental disorder not only may her condition make necessary restraint in bed by straps or sheets, but the windows of the room should be barred.

Postoperative management depends very largely upon the type of operation performed. As a rule those carried out by the abdominal route are classed as major procedures and those by the vaginal route as minor. The subject may, therefore, best be considered in its application to one or the other of these routes.

## ABDOMINAL SECTION

*Pain.*—During the first twenty-four hours after operation the patient suffers from pain in greater or lesser degree. At times this pain is limited to the wound but oftener it is due to tension, when the parietal peritoneum is involved, as in ventrosuspension, or when the broad ligaments are pulled upon, as in round ligament shortening. More pain is experienced in the lateral, muscle-splitting incision than in the median wound, through the linea alba. When the pain is not so severe as to produce restlessness or wakefulness the patient is better without a narcotic, but this is rarely the case, and sufficient sedative must be given to prevent the exhaustion and depression subsequent to severe or prolonged suffering. Morphin sulphate (grn. 1/8 to 1/6) is given during the first night, usually at once after operation, since the pain is then at its worse. While morphin favors distention, thus tending to unsettle the stomach, flatulence seldom appears until twenty-four hours after operation. Peritonitis and intestinal obstruction, which are masked by morphin, rarely develop until after forty-eight hours. Morphin is never given by routine but only as each dose is specifically prescribed and, in any case, if prolonged is most undesirable. Heroin (grn. 1/2 to 1/6) alone or combined with pyramidon (grn. v.) provides a satisfactory substitute in ordinarily severe cases. This may be given every eight hours for three days following operation.

After the pain of trauma has passed or been allayed, morphin is contraindicated, distress now being due to intestinal colic for which free evacuation of the colon and rectum is the treatment. Neurotic patients will complain of great pain and show extreme restlessness, though pulse and temperature are normal and distention is absent. Morphin here is particularly to be avoided, anodynes being of as much value. Where the pain during the first day is out of proportion to the nature of the operation and to the temperament of the patient, especially if the pulse is unduly rapid, some trouble at the operation site is to be suspected. Pain unduly severe after forty-eight hours is the result of distention, peritonitis, or intestinal obstruction.

As regards the ordinary gas pains, so common after abdominal section, they indicate activity on the part of the bowel, particularly of the small intestine. Nothing is so ominous as an absolute absence of pain or distress at once after operation, a condition strongly suggective of shock and paralytic ileus. While no surgeon wants his patient to suffer unduly, the appearance of the well-recognized gas pain at least means that the bowel is active. Accompanied by the passage of flatus, the abdomen remaining soft, this is a fortunate sign, and contraindicates, rather than demands, much medication.

Relief from pain is not so urgent and often not required when the operation has been preceded by the administration of an opiate. Morphin and atropin prior to operation was for years a routine practice and remains the routine with many surgeons. In the practice of others the combination of morphin and scopolamin, the "twilight sleep" of obstetrics, is employed and constitutes the main feature of the surgical anesthesia. Operators employing methods of local anesthesia also often precede those by scopolamin-morphin narcosis. Naturally, in methods such as these, with whatever variable and elastic changes they may be modified, postoperative analgesic treatment is reduced to a minimum.

With the perfection of gas-ether administration, and particularly in cases in which nitrous oxid gas or ethylene gas may be used without ether, all preliminary narcosis is best omitted and atropin is unnecessary. In my practice the administration of nitrous oxid or ethylene gas, with or without ether, has become the method of choice, and the postoperative use of morphin sulphate or heroin hydrochlorate is not only desirable but necessary. Given at this time the drug is employed in the minimum dosage essential to the relief of pain, its one and only indication.

Restlessness or insomnia may persist at times without a continuance of pain, and in such cases physiological methods of treatment are often sufficient. A sponge bath, a change in the patient's position in bed, gentle massage, a pillow under the knees, are small things which serve to induce sleep or bring about composure. Sleeplessness is seen without pain in various patients, especially if exposed to the disturbing influences of the large ward. Here again, is an argument for the isolation ward following laparotomy. For the patient who is restless through sheer anxiety or nervousness, no drugs are more effective than the bromids, occasionally with the addition of chloral. Persistent insomnia is a sign often preceding or accompanying peritonitis, intestinal obstruction, and postoperative insanity. It is also a result of toxic absorption, as from the operation area. The ability to sleep readily after operation gives excellent prognosis for a speedy and uneventful convalescence.

*Emesis.*—While regarded as due chiefly to the anesthetic, vomiting occurs more frequently after abdominal sections than after operation on other parts of the body. Hence it results in part from invasion of the peritoneal cavity, handling of the intestines, and extirpation of organs inverted with peritoneum. While ether is, without doubt, the most generally employed anesthetic agent, there is an evident advantage in the use of gas-ether combinations. Not only does the patient awaken more speedily, but vomiting is definitely decreased. In short and relatively superficial operations, making possible nitrous oxid-oxygen or ethylene gas-oxygen anesthesia, no vomiting at all occurs in a fairly large proportion of cases. It is less persistent and less violent, if present at all, when little or no ether is employed, as in the preoperative morphin-scopolamin narcosis or in local anesthesia, by infiltration, nerve blocking, intraspinal, and like methods. It should be noted as well, that patients poorly prepared for operation, or those acutely ill and suffering from emesis prior to operation, will have more after-distress. Speed of work, handling tissues gently, avoiding the intestine as much as possible, limiting the field of manipulation to the pathologic area, and like measures in technic have their importance from the prophylactic point of view.

In the routine work of the clinic, however, there will be that series of cases in which the anesthetic must be profound, for deep pelvic work, extensive enucleation, or careful peritoneal toilet, and in which ether is the only means of securing relaxation and exposure. In such cases postoperative vomiting is anticipated and usually experienced. This was formerly regarded as a symptom of gastric catarrh and Herman taught that the stomach should be kept empty, a treatment difficult to carry out because of the patient's thirst. Ashton has advocated oxygen inhalation until consciousness begins to return, when vinegar is substituted until the patient is awake. Anesthetic vomiting rarely lasts more than a few hours, but when gastritis has been produced, it may be prolonged for a day—the "irritative" form of Bomey and not associated with untoward symptoms such as fever, rapid pulse, or abdominal rigidity.

Neurotic patients often display the most intractable vomiting, cases in which there is little or no reason to suspect any grave intra-abdominal lesion, and in which all methods of treatment are of no avail. The amount of fluid expelled does not increase and the only harm is that food is not taken or retained. Occasionally the vomiting ceases for no apparent reason, and often the employment of some unusual artifice will suffice. Placing an ice-bag over the epigastrium, or a weak mustard paste may serve the purpose. A small amount of brandy in hot water taken at once after emesis is at times successful in alleviating further difficulty. In prolonged cases all food is stopped by mouth and nutrient enemata are given after colonic flushing and gastric lavage. The latter procedure is often sufficient in itself. Washing out the stomach with a tube may so distress a neurotic patient that there will be no further emesis.

The most effective measures, were it not for excessive thirst, would be to keep the stomach empty and to flush the colon with soapsuds enemata. But fluid taken by mouth, especially if cold, is often retained, accumulating in quantity until vomited. Undoubtedly the most distressing nausea is that in which the stomach is relatively empty, containing but a small amount of its own secretions. Lavage in such cases is the most effective treatment but, since the passing of a tube is in itself distressing, the same end is attained by having the patient drink hot water. If nausea without vomiting is present, hot water in teaspoonful doses is given every few minutes. But as long as the patient vomits she is encouraged to drink hot water freely, in as large amount as she can be made to take. If vomited it comes up easily, without the retching and gagging so often seen years ago. The stomach is then quiet for a time and eventually the water is retained, the stomach is washed out downward, and then sodium bicarbonate is given in half-teaspoonful doses with each subsequent glass of water.

After vomiting has ceased food is given at once. As a rule liquids are well taken, but some solid food, such as egg-albumin and toast with tea, in small quantities, is of greater value. After the first bowel movement soft food is allowed. In the absence of flatulence milk and milk foods are given.

When nausea and vomiting have continued beyond forty-eight hours, evidences of peritonitis are sought.

*Thirst.*—After a major operation the first complaint of the patient upon awakening is often that of thirst. This is due to loss of fluid by free perspiration during operation, to the loss of blood and serum incident to the operation, and it is probably, in some degree, one expression of reaction to the physical assault of operation. When atropin has been administered as a pre-operative measure there results a dryness of the throat, giving the patient the sensation of thirst. This has not been a factor in my practice during recent years, since gas-oxygen or ether-gas-oxygen anesthesia has been employed, preceding which morphin and atropin are not given. Thirst is prevented, therefore, by the copious ingestion of water during the day or two prior to operation, and by the administration of a pint of tap water, or normal salt solution, per rectum at once after the patient is returned to bed. Thereafter six ounces of saline is injected every few hours.

As soon as the nausea ceases and hot water taken by mouth is retained there is no further complaint of thirst. The water should not be given warm, which is unpleasant to many people, but as hot as tea is ordinarily drunk, so that it may be sipped from the spoon. Cold water, or chipped ice, may be more refreshing in the mouth, but it does not allay thirst so well and is more apt to induce accumulation in the stomach, being actually harmful if flatulence coexists. During the entire convalescence the patient is encouraged to drink freely of water, especially the still mineral varieties.

When the patient is definitely toxic, or when, as in the case of prolonged inflammatory disease, such as chronic pelvic peritonitis, acidosis may ensue after operation, the enemata are alkalinized, or combined with glucose solution. Bicarbonate of soda is given by mouth as soon as hot water is retained. In some of these cases it which the patients are badly run down, a preoperative carbohydrate feeding is well indicated, together with the elimination from the diet of meat and eggs for a period of several days. After operation, instead of the normal saline solution every four hours, a solution of malt sugar or 20 per cent dextromaltose is substituted. This is continued for several days, or until the urine is only slightly acid. This method of alkalinization not only tends to prevent or overcome thirst, but has a definite influence upon nausea, distention, and the healing of the wound.

*Temperature, Pulse, Respiration.*—The rate of the pulse and respiration and the degree of temperature are taken and recorded by the nurse every six hours during the first ten days, and twice daily thereafter in the absence of complications. If the patient is too restless, or is hysterical or unconscious, the *temperature* is taken more accurately by the bowel. As a rule fever does not rise above 101° or 102° F., often not exceeding 100° F. This post-operative rise is highest on the second day, thereafter dropping to 99° F., becoming normal after the bowels are evacuated. A temperature maintained at 99° or 100° F. for a week has no especial significance, but a rise after the bowels have moved suggests beginning suppuration in the wound or a circumscribed peritoneal infection. Persistently high temperature indicates a stitch-abscess in the abdominal wound, especially if associated with local pain or soreness. Nervousness, worry, or the annoyance of too many visitors often causes a sudden rise of fever, which is not maintained but subsides with rest.

Quite the most satisfactory guide with respect to the patient's condition after operation is the *pulse*. As a rule its course is high or low proportionately with the temperature. Its rate does not go beyond 100 during the first three days of normal convalescence, and declines after bowel elimination. During the first twenty-four hours the pulse rate varies according to the length of the operation, its character, the amount of blood lost, and factors of such kind. The anesthetic and pre-operative narcosis also has its influence, the pulse being slowed down if scopolamin or like drugs have been given. For this reason, as an indication of actual conditions the pulse is most reliable, again, when ether-gas or gas-oxygen anesthesia has been employed.

In the normal case the pulse should run about 80, full, even, regular, and soft. An increase at this time, following free catharsis, is indicative of infection, especially if coincident with some fever and abdominal tympany or rigidity. A rate of 115 to 130 after the second day shows a serious condition, while a rate of 140 goes without signs of shock or hemorrhage. In hysteria or other states of excitation the rate is increased temporarily.

Rapid *respiration* soon after operation indicates shock or hemorrhage; later it is associated with peritonitis, intestinal obstruction or pulmonary complication. With much abdominal pain the patient breathes more superficially and hence with a slightly increased rate. After the second day, or upon the cessation of vomiting, respiration becomes relatively normal, full, deep, rhythmical, varying slightly about 20 to the minute.

*The Mouth and Tongue.*—Frequent cleansing of the mouth is a grateful relief to the patient, the nurse using a cool solution of boric acid or a modified Dobell's. Artificial teeth are not restored until vomiting has definitely ceased. A soft toothbrush is employed as soon as the patient has recovered sufficient strength. The tongue shows characteristic changes according to conditions. After the first day it is moist but remains white as long as the diet is liquid. In the severer forms of infection or obstruction, particularly with fever, it becomes dry and brown, fissured and red, or ulcerated. In such case the lips become chapped or fissured and require annointing frequently with olive oil or a bland ointment.

*The Diet.*—Feeding by mouth should not be attempted until the stomach is quiet. By our modern methods of anesthesia, however, emesis is often absent and seldom prolonged. Hence the ingestion of food may be started early. For the first twenty-four hours after operation the patient will most probably have no desire to eat, but if she does she may be given egg-albumin, beef juice, or weak tea, and, in some instances, even a slice of buttered toast. After the first bowel evacuation soft diet is given, light diet by the fifth or sixth day, and the full tray substituted for the second week. Milk is best omitted, particularly during the stay in bed, as it increases flatulence and may prolong nausea and vomiting. Milk is a solid food after its ingestion and must be used with discretion. As a rule it is best taken in a peptonized form or with lime water. It is also acceptable in the form of cooked foods, such as puddings and custards.

Orange or grape juice, unsweetened, is agreeable as soon as liquids can be retained. Alcoholic stimulants are given only on definite indication and have a certain value, the best forms being brandy, sherry, or champagne. Formerly we gave an ounce of whisky added to the first retention enema, as a routine. A wine glass of sherry, two or three times daily, after the first week, may be given with value for a few weeks after operation.

Where the operative procedures have involved the intestinal tract, as in appendectomy, the dietary as outlined is to be advanced somewhat more cautiously, any considerable amount of food, and all solids, being withheld during the first three or four days. On the other hand, prolonged gastric distress, not due to some actual complications, does not contraindicate solid food, many patients doing better as soon as liquid diet is discontinued. After regular diet is in order, nourishing liquids, such as hot chocolate, malted milk, egg-nog and fruit juice, are offered between meals.

Again it is worth while to emphasize the importance of alkalinization and glucose proctoclysis as a means of preventing or combating acidosis. This may exist, unsuspected, before operation and be the cause of prolonged emesis after, or it may follow as the result of vomiting. The essential element lies in the deflection of the alkali reserve in the blood, and starvation acidosis must be counteracted before any hope can be entertained of establishing food balance. It is claimed by some that acetone formed as the result of the action of ether upon the organism together with the by-products of a rich protein diet following operation, are responsible for many postoperative discomforts, even for faulty wound healing. Hence the preoperative feeding of milk sugar and sodium bicarbonate instead of milk and eggs and the continuance of soda and glucose solutions after operation, as has been previously outlined.

*Management of the Urinary Tract.*—This constitutes one of the most important features of postoperative care. After abdominal section most patients are able to void spontaneously, but such a large proportion required some assistance in this respect, and infection of the bladder is a complication so distressing and so potentially dangerous that every measure should be taken to avoid it. According to Curtis, 66 per cent of his patients subjected to major gynecological operations required no catheterization, 11 per cent required it once, 5 per cent required it twice and 17 per cent required it three or more times. Mills' report shows that of 321 abdominal operations upon the pelvic organs, 145 patients, 45 per cent required catheterization. Mills also found that women are more liable to bladder disturbances than men, as is shown by the figures in one group of 420 patients, male and female, in which the operations and treatment were the same. In this group, 3.1 per cent of the men and 23.1 per cent of the women required catheterization.

In the case of that patient who does not void spontaneously, effort is made to induce urination every eight hours. Micturition is encouraged by local hot applications, by steaming water poured into the bed-pan, by external douching with warm water, and such methods. The application to the urinary meatus of some stimulating substance, such as a drop of spirits of camphor, is employed successfully at times. The best form of diuresis consists in increasing the amount of fluid to be excreted by the normal saline enemata previously referred to and by the copious drinking of hot water. Eventually the patient is allowed to go four more hours before catheterizing her. In other words, attempts at inducing urination are made every eight hours, catheterization every twelve hours. As in postpartum convalescence, a patient finds it difficult to void while lying on her back; conditions permitting, it is better to support her in a sitting or reclining position on the bed-pan than to use the catheter. Where the ability to void naturally is once regained it is apt to be retained regardless of position. Occasionally, too, a patient is unable to void spontaneously as long as she is confined to bed but does so without difficulty at once upon arising. Again, nervous irritability and bladder difficulties are commonly associated.

The first specimen voided after operation, or obtained by the catheter, is sent to the laboratory. After that, analysis is made only as may be indicated by special conditions, though twice weekly is not too often as a routine. The total excretion is diminished during the first three days and more or less vesical irritability is occasioned as a result of concentration. Hence it may be advisable to measure and record the total daily output.

Emphasis must always be placed upon the technic of surgical cleanliness in the use of the catheter. This need not be detailed here but the nurse should have adequate assistance in the performance of such a procedure which, though minor technically, is of major importance. Assistance is invariably necessary when the patient is unconscious, is struggling from nervousness, pain or hysteria, or when she is delirious. In some cases the urinary meatus is difficult to find. Then the head nurse, or the resident or attending surgeon, is called.

For a long time it has been believed that postoperative cystitis results from infection due to imperfect technic in catheterization. To-day such infection is regarded as secondary to the contamination of residual urine. Of the 66 per cent of patients in his series in whom the use of the catheter was unnecessary, Curtis found residual urine in less than 1 per cent. But of the 17 per cent, 269 patients, requiring catheterization three or more times, residual urine was found in 64 per cent. The amount of this residual retention decreases gradually as the bladder regains its power of complete evacuation, a period usually varying from four to eight days.

According to the present plan of treatment the catheter is used for the relief of distention, rarely oftener than every twelve hours. If this has occurred more than three times the patient is catheterized daily immediately after one urination and this is continued until the residual urine has disappeared, or is less than one ounce and free from pus. During this time the urine is rendered acid by sodium acetate, and hexamethylenamin is given in quantities sufficient to reveal free formaldehyd. After each catheterization one or two ounces of silver nitrate solution (1-3000) may be left in the bladder, particularly if the hexamethylenamin is omitted. After plastic operations involving the bladder itself the test catheterization for residual retention is advisable for a few days even if the patient is voiding spontaneously. Furthermore, it is unwise to stop suddenly the use of the catheter when micturition becomes spontaneous, for the reason that the bladder is usually unable to empty itself completely for several more days. The residual urine, thus accumulating, becomes contaminated and gives rise to cystitis, the same as it does in the first instance.

*Management of the Bowels.*—The postoperative care of the bowels depends largely upon preoperative preparation. At the present day it is generally understood that catharsis beginning the day before abdominal section, particularly that intestinal evacuation formerly described as "thorough," does more harm than good. It causes the patient to have a disturbed and restless night, it produces psychic and physical weakness, loss of body and intestinal fluids, change in the bacterial flora of the bowel with hypertonicity of its wall, and irritability of rectum and colon. The postoperative thirst is greater and the gas pains are more marked. To-day drastic purgation as a preparation for operation has been abandoned. A mild laxative the night before and an enema the morning of the operation is regarded as sufficient in many clinics. In others a laxative is given two days before and an enema the evening before. A few surgeons continue the purge and enema before operation, others have come to omit all except the enema and a few object even to it.

The old time system of pre-operative starvation has also been discontinued. A light meal the evening before, or fluids only, may be wiser in anticipation of surgical procedure involving the gastro-intestinal tract directly; but for gynecological operations this is less important, and the omission of the meal preceding the anesthetic is, in most cases, sufficient. As food leaves the small intestine within twelve hours after taking, nothing is gained by withholding it—if easily digested and in moderate quantity—up to this time. It is desirable, in lower abdominal procedures, to have the colon empty and, hence, a high enema shortly before operation will suffice.

In considering the treatment of emesis and pain the use of the enema was discussed. Its value, then, is rather from this point of view and from that of evacuation of the bowel. Hence, purgation need seldom be hurried, but may usually be put off until after the third day. Where the stomach is unsettled, little is gained by giving cathartics by mouth. Some authorities prescribe calomel in divided doses as early as forty-eight hours after operation, following it by enemata of soapsuds and glycerin. Others employ magnesium sulphate or castor oil by the end of the second day if the stomach is settled, with an enema to follow up turpentine and soapsuds.

On the contrary, certain authors in the more recent literature argue against the postoperative cathartic. Thus, Taylor and his associates report interesting observations in the care of a large series of patients. They divided these into three groups: (1) those purged before and after operation, (2) those not purged before but purged shortly after, and (3) those not purged before and who were given no enema or cathartic for at least four days after operation. The omission of the pre-operative purge had no definite influence on the vomiting but reduced pain from 75 per cent to 42 per cent. Delay in giving the postoperative purge reduced emesis from 45 per cent to 30 per cent. In both groups complaint of pain was greater when the postoperative purges and enemas were withheld. Howard gave a postoperative cathartic in the treatment of 200 cases of peritonitis, and obtained better results by thus allowing the patient to remain quiet than he had secured previously by the routine use of calomel. The tendency to give cathartics too soon after abdominal section is also deplored by Bell who relies chiefly on the enema. As soon as peristalsis is once well started it usually continues actively, so that simple laxative, such as cascara sagrada, or podophyllin, or the aloin-belladonna pill, are not required during the patient's stay in bed.

While most women are chronically constipated, some are not and these latter will reveal as much distress during the second and third weeks from ordinary laxatives, for instance, as they do at once after operation. Routine treatment is essential in hospital practice, especially in the larger wards, yet the routine should be so flexible as to be readily adjusted to the individual requirement of each patient. In most cases this adjustment is toward repeated efforts to overcome chronic intestinal stasis, particularly that type aggravated by the mechanical sagging and developmental loss of tone characterizing enteroptosis. In such a case, postsurgical, repeated enemata are required, soap and water, containing an ounce of glycerin or a half ounce of turpentine, or, glycerin and sweet oil combined, placed as high in the colon as possible by means of a long tube. The treatment, however, is for the immediate convalescence only. As soon as conditions allow that food be taken, treatment of the spastic constipation is begun by a carefully formulated dietary. It is always best if the patient can be well started on this plan before leaving the hospital.

It has been shown by Soper that, in the type of patient under discussion, spastic contractures of the lower colon and rectum play an important part in the etiology of chronic constipation and, as well, of postoperative gas pains and abdominal distention. Soper advises that this condition be treated by the injection through the rectal tube of three ounces of a saturated solution of magnesium sulphate, with the hips elevated in order to promote as long a retention as possible. This is repeated every day or several times daily, with no signs of toxicity when the enema was retained as long as twenty-four hours.

During the early postoperative days the colon tube is of definite value as a means of relieving the patient of flatus. Postoperative distention is one of the first conditions calling for treatment and has been discussed in previous paragraphs. Tympany rarely appears before the second day and, if there is any delay in the expulsion of gas, or if the abdomen is seen to be distending, the colon tube is passed at once. It may be passed several times a day and may be left in the bowel for a half hour or so at a time. In this way flatus is expelled readily, without the painful bearing-down effort on the part of the patient, an effort, indeed, which she often will not make because of pain, or cannot make because of muscular trauma. Aid in the expulsion of gas is lent by strychnin sulphate (grn. 1/20) or an ampule of pituitrin, injected hypodermically. Pituitrin is particularly effective in the more obstinate forms of simple distention, in paralytic ileus, and in the cases already referred to as characterized by muscular insufficiency and ptosis. Eserin salicylate (grn.

1/40) is always mentioned in this connection, and is highly regarded by many writers. Stevens uses it in association with digitalis (grn. 1/50) and strychnin sulphate (grn. 1/60). Eserin has proved of little value in my experience. On the contrary pituitrin is very helpful in its limited field. Its influence is temporary, so that it may be required in repeated doses. In pathological hypertension it is contraindicated as it is in intestinal obstruction and ileus due to peritonitis.

*Care of the Wound.*—When the wound is closed as described in Section VI, page 200, it is left untouched until the fifth day when the gauze roll beneath the retention sutures may be removed. Then, if the abdomen is soft and flat, the sutures may be retired. In case of abdominal distention the roll had better be left in place. Indeed, it is not necessary that the roll be removed and the wound may be left untouched until time for removal of the stitches. When the superficial skin drain, such as is advantageously placed in the obese abdominal wall, has been used, this is withdrawn on the second day, not later than the third, again necessitating change of dressings. Aside from these exceptions the wound is not disturbed unless there is fever, pain in the wound, or the dressing is soaked with blood or other discharging fluids. In redressing fresh gauze is used throughout, the original adhesive strips being replaced by short straps, adherent laterally and tied together over the dressing by tapes.

Some experienced surgeons seal the wound with strips of gauze bandage and collodion, and this is covered, in turn, with several layers of gauze and adhesive plaster. After five or six hours the outer dressing is removed and an ice bag is placed over the wound for the purpose of allaying pain. The sealed wound heals very well in case of the thin abdominal wall. In the few cases requiring drainage, however, this dressing is impossible and in case of the fat wall, where the wound juices often ooze for two or three days, the collodion-gauze dressing serves only to retain these discharges. Free drainage is one of the best assurances of primary and sound healing. In past years I have covered the wound with a four-layer gauze dressing, sealing its edges only with collodion, so that the incision itself remained covered, but unsealed. Even with this method the gauze would become clogged with secretions in the obese patient. At the present the gauze roll is regarded as most satisfactory, though this may be sealed at the lower angle of the wound in order to keep the incision from being exposed to infection from below when the patient flexes her legs, thus causing the binder and other dressings to gape. Over any dressing there may be placed the ice-bag which relieves the pain in the wound but has no influence upon gas pains, as has been claimed by some.

In general hospital routine, the average laparotomy dressing is too abundant. Only enough gauze should be used to assure the wound protection from contamination, never keeping it hot and moist. For the same reason wet antiseptic dressings, formerly advocated by certain experienced operators, have no place in the clean surgical field.

The superficial skin stitches are removed on the seventh or eighth day, the deeper retention ones on the tenth day. In the dressing that has been undisturbed the deeper layers of gauze are apt to be adherent along the edges of the wound and these are more readily freed if first soaked by hydrogen peroxid. The wound is sponged with alcohol, after removal of the stitches, and fresh dressings applied, with the scultetus binder over all.

*Wound Infection.*—One of the most annoying incidents of convalescence is infection of the wound. While slight infection is of relatively little importance it may lead to grave complications, and, in any event, it spoils what may be otherwise a technically perfect and therapeutically successful operation. It is due to contamination from septic tissues below, from the skin surface of the abdomen, or to technical faults at the time of operation, less often to imperfectly sterilized suture material. Imperfect hemostasis, giving rise to subcutaneous hematoma which are ideal culture media, or the retention of broken-down fat globules or of serum may be the factors. In anemia, debilitated patients, as those suffering from carcinoma, tuberculosis, and sometimes lues, the process of healing is retarded and less resistance is offered to infection.

Stitch abscess appears, as a rule, on the sixth or eighth day, though it may not occur until after the stitches have been removed. The reaction is altogether local, often with not enough pain and soreness in the wound to attract attention. Sometimes the abscess is discovered at the first postoperative dressing. In other cases more than one stitch may be involved and, by the time discovered, a portion of the wound has become undermined by an accumulation of pus. The local symptoms are then more severe, with a rise of temperature and onset of pain and soreness locally. The possibility of stitch abscess should be borne in mind constantly and the slightest symptoms suggesting it must be investigated. Early recognition and treatment are necessary to prevent a slight infection from extending into a general suppuration.

When the entire abdominal wound breaks down, the abscess usually forms in the subcutaneous fat, the pus swelling towards the surface between the stitches and forcing apart the edges of the wound to greater or less extent. Only rarely do the interrupted stitches uniting the fascia become involved, in which case the entire wound will open as far as the peritoneum. Even here the tendency is to point upward, and only in exceptional cases has rupture occurred into the peritoneal cavity. Symptoms of wound suppuration appear by the end of the first week or middle of the second. The temperature is irregular, septic in type, but higher than it should be at this stage of convalescence. The pulse is correspondingly accelerated. Discomfort in the wound is at first noticed; later it becomes acutely painful and tender. Inspection shows indurated wound edges which are fluctuant to palpation if abscess formation has taken place. The dressings are apt to be stained or already soaked with the discharging material.

When suppuration has involved the fascial and muscular layers, symptoms of septicemia suddenly develop and these continue progressively until the wound discharges spontaneously or is treated. Septic peritonitis, with violent reaction and the speedy collapse of the patient, may ensue even without actual rupture of the peritoneum.

The integrity of the wound is impaired little or not at all, if the infectious process is limited to the subcutaneous space. On the contrary, danger of subsequent hernia naturally is present if the deeper lines of suture become involved. The length of the wound is of some importance also, as is the extent of lateral burrowing by the pus. As a rule these infections tend to clear up promptly when treated, the wound closing by granulation and cicatrization from below. An important factor, as well, in the prognosis is the general condition of the patient.

In the prophylaxis of wound infection more depends upon the technical details of operation than anything else. Certain of these have been emphasized in earlier sections of this volume and need but be mentioned again. The wound is prepared for closure at the time it is made, thus avoiding fresh bleeding when ready for closure. The wound edges are protected by folding the towels or sheets about them and including these in the grasp of the retractor blades. The wound is sufficiently long to accommodate the operator to the exigencies of the procedure being carried out, so that wound edges are not subjected to prolonged strain or undue pressure. Infected material is removed from the abdominal cavity in such a way as to leave the freshly incised walls uncontaminated.

Before closing, all bleeding points are securely ligated. Closure is effected by suturing in layers, in order not to leave dead spaces for the accumulation of blood, serum, or fat. Non-absorbable suture material is to be avoided if it must be buried. The skin edges are not continuously approximated, as when closed by subcuticular suture, because this prevents seepage from the wound. In thick abdominal walls suppuration is more liable to occur and greater care is exercised in order to prevent dead spaces. An extra layer of catgut may be run through the subcutaneous fat, and this fat must not be undercut too much, else the formation of a dead space is inevitable. Preferable to this is a slender drain of gutta percha or rubber tissue, or a few strands of silkworm gut, placed just beneath the skin and long enough to protrude at either end. After the skin stitches are in, the wound area is cleansed with alcohol, the retention sutures are tied over a gauze roll, and, over all, the dressings are applied.

The treatment of wound infection should be prompt and active. As soon as local inflammation is suspected the dressings are removed for inspection. If redness or induration is present, or if a stitch abscess has formed, hot wet dressings (of boric acid solution) are applied. These are kept on continuously until induration and excessive redness disappear. No sutures are removed, no drains inserted, and the wound is not probed. According to the experience of Watkins, who has advocated this method of treatment for many years, no appreciable cavity is present at the site of suppuration and intraabdominal and atmospheric pressure keep the discharging surfaces in relative apposition. When drainage ceases no open wound exists. Under this régime infected wounds heal more promptly, patients are less disturbed, and the abdominal wall is left much stronger than after the more energetic treatment formerly in vogue.

In those occasional cases in which the wound opens, to a greater or less extent throughout its length, the hot wet dressings are continued, and irrigation, if required at all, is best effected with the hypochlorite solutions. The wound may be poured full of dichloramin-T in solution, the dressings being changed twice daily, if the patient must remain on her back. Drains are unnecessary and if she is made to lie on the side or in the lateroprone position, discharging material will not be retained. As a rule Sims' position and hot wet dressings are all that is essential to speedy filling in and closure of the wound. With the appearance of clean granulations the adhesive straps are tightened and the gaping edges brought into approximation. If granulation tissue fills in in excess, it is curetted away and the skin margins, slightly undercut and trimmed, are brought together again as in the original closure.

When the suppurative focus is limited to the subcutaneous tissue, the patient's stay in bed need not be prolonged beyond the regular time demanded by her case. It is not, however, advisable to discharge her from the hospital with a discharging wound.

*Sinus tracts* complicating the healing of abdominal wounds are rarely seen in these days when absorbable suture material is more extensively employed than formerly and more adequately prepared. The disuse of drainage, once so common, is another factor and, a third, careful peritonization of stumps and pedicle ligatures deep in the pelvis. These tracts in many respects resemble fistulous ones but there is absent the characteristic escape of feces or urine. A probe will pass to the bottom of the sinus where a somewhat extensive cavity may be determined or where other tracts lead off to other foci of infection. The spontaneous discharge of an infected non-absorbable suture is a matter of months and should not be awaited. Little is gained by probing or attempting to locate the offending suture with a snare.

In the certain absence of a foreign body a sinus might be effectively closed by infiltrating it with bismuth paste; otherwise expectant treatment is no longer the established method of dealing with these cases. Where the tract is extraperitoneal an incision is made through the old scar, the infected sinus is dissected out, or curetted free from necrotic tissue, and the wound allowed to close in from below.

Temporizing treatment of a sinus leading into the pelvis is usually futile, and operation is indicated. With a long probe introduced along the tract, the abdomen is cautiously opened and the adherent intestinal coils freed carefully until the bottom of the tract is located. Every effort is made to dissect the sinus throughout its entire extent before attempting removal, as it is extremely difficult to extirpate such an area piecemeal. The greatest danger is in injury to the intestine which is invariably convoluted and plastered about the tract, and often nothing but a tubulated mass of adhesions. After removal of the sinus the abdomen should be closed without drainage if possible.

*Urinary fistula,* when due to ureteral injury, has been discussed in Section VI. Injury to the bladder usually closes spontaneously but in rare instances this fails and leaking persists. In the one case which I have seen of this sort, the failure of vesical closure was apparently due to a loop of the ileum which had become adherent to the parietal peritoneum and to the bladder just below the point of injury. In this case the abdomen was reopened, the bowel freed, the bladder mobilized and its wound repaired, and the abdomen then closed without drainage, although a retention catheter was passed through the urethra.

*Fecal fistulæ,* following abdominal operations, occur when there has been injury to the intestinal coats entailed in separating adhesions, when a portion of the intestinal wall has become necrotic from contact with an inflammatory mass, or when an injury has been repaired or anastomosis performed with subsequent leakage. The great majority of fistulæ follow the removal of pus tubes, especially if these are tuberculous in nature and the adhesions, therefore, extremely dense, intimate, and extensive. Rarely, fistula is due to infection in the abdominal wall, a coil of intestine having become adherent beneath and later necrotic. Necrosis due to the pressure of drainage material, especially glass or rubber tubing, has been known also to result in a fistula.

The proportion of fistulæ involving the colon, invariably the sigmoid flexure or cecum, close spontaneously, as a rule. Closure is hastened if the patient is kept on a diet of concentrated foods, operation rarely becoming necessary. The small intestine adherent to the abdominal wall produces a fistula of more serious import. The contents being liquid and more irritating to the skin, spontaneous closure is delayed, though it does take place. If the upper portion of the bowel is involved, general emaciation due to loss of food increases the gravity of the situation.

As soon as the patient's condition makes it possible, a permanent fistula should be closed. As a rule this is best done not later than three months after the original operation by which time the scar is well organized and recent granulation tissue no longer present. Incision is made parallel to the old wound but not too close, in order to avoid adhesions, if possible, upon opening the peritoneum. From within the adherent loop of bowel is then carefully forced and the extent of the injury to its coat investigated. If the hole is a small one it is closed by a purse-string of fine catgut. Sometimes the wound is linear and is then repaired by an over-and-over whip-stitch, care being taken to close it in such a way as not to restrict unduly the lumen of the bowel. Resection with end-to-end or lateral anastomosis is rarely indicated —only when there is extensive loss of continuity of the gut, as in dense infiltration, gangrene, or obstruction. Lateral anastomosis without resection, merely short-circuiting the fistula, or colostomy above the fistula, are almost equally extensive procedures without certainty of cure.

# SYMPTOMS IN GYNECOLOGY

ISIDOR CLINTON RUBIN, M.D.

## APPENDIX

### THE IMPORTANCE OF A UNIFORM PRESSURE RATE FLOW IN TRANS-UTERINE INSUFFLATION TO DETERMINE PATENCY OF THE FALLOPIAN TUBES

The method of transuterine insufflation first devised in 1919 has been widely adopted and is employed not only by the specialist in gynecology but also by the general practitioner. The test of tubal patency has developed out of many attempts to find a method simple enough to be employed as a routine diagnostic procedure similar, let us say, to cystoscopy. I have done transuterine insufflation many hundreds of times in my office either alone or with the assistance of one nurse. Yet notwithstanding this uncomplicated technic there have been a not inconsiderable number of modifications of the method whose purpose was still further to simplify the original method. It has been held that the apparatus required is too cumbersome, necessitating the assistance of one or two persons. For the convenience of others I adopted the automatically acting siphon volumeter to which has been added a manometer (Fig. 1). The apparatus is not cumbersome. The outlay made at the beginning is permanent and except for refilling the gas tank needs a negligible amount of handling.

The fact that carbon dioxid has proved to be the most readily resorbed of all the available gases has made it preferable for use in the office. The commercial supply of this gas is usually delivered in large quantities and under great pressure requiring therefore a reduction valve to regulate its flow.

There are two ways by which this cumbersome reduction-valve factor can be removed. One is by means of the "sparklets" used in some places to charge water for drinking purposes. Unfortunately the amount of gas contained in the sparklet is not adequate for prolonged use, and unless one has need for daily use of the test one has to change the sparklets each time. It requires a special attachment and a special reduction valve entailing the trouble of frequent replacement. When the sparklet is used the outflow of the gas being regulated by the reduction valve, it delivers a uniform flow of carbon dioxid gas in a manner satisfactory for our purposes.

Another plan is to transfer the gas from the large tank to a smaller tank without a reduction valve as is ordinarily employed in gas anesthesia. Such a smaller tank can be easily fastened to the examining table in the manner illustrated below, and within a few minutes at stated intervals the tank can be refilled when the gas is reduced to low ebb and low pressure. This method is one which I have used and find it satisfactory as it ensures in the best possible way a uniform flow of the gas under a constant pressure rate. If oxygen is used it may be taken from the tanks in ordinary commmercial use; those with a fine valve and circular handle (not a small lever) are preferable. I have used this method in several hundred cases and have found it most serviceable. Once the apparatus is assembled, the actual operation in the method of transuterine insufflation may be controlled by a single examiner.

Many references have been made to the necessity of having one or more assistants during the procedure, and the uterine cannula has been modified in a number of ways, some even devising self-retaining instruments

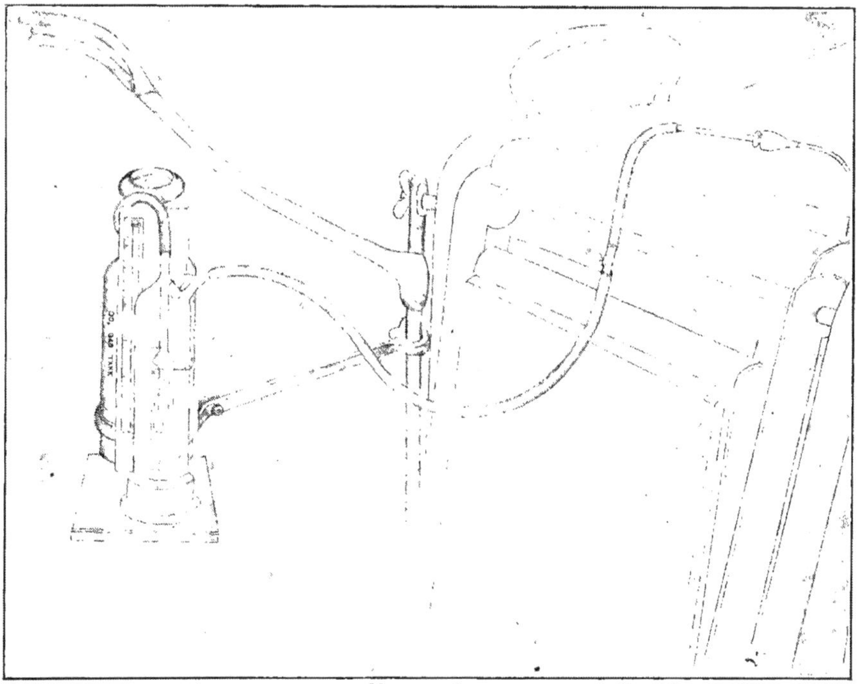

FIG. 1.—AUTHOR'S APPARATUS FOR UTERINE INSUFFLATION TO TEST TUBAL PATENCY.

so as to liberate one hand of the examiner for other purposes. In the technic as employed by those of us who have started with the method from its early inception the cannula and bullet forceps may be handled by one hand while the other hand is free for other purposes. I have on many occasions introduced the cannula into the uterus and left the cannula and bullet forceps resting on the lower leaf of the speculum without steadying either during the insufflation thus leaving both hands free. In my hands it has seemed to be a very satisfactory, simple procedure requiring no extra assistance.

A number of modifications have been made of the test, practically all of them calculated to simplify the "Rubin test." Thus the record syringe varying in capacity from 20 to 150 c.c. has been used by different operators. Others prefer the rubber bulb with a metal cannula or with a glass cannula either of which is provided with one outflow and no manometer or with a T-shaped branch to which a manometer is attached. In this apparatus naturally air is the medium employed. When the record syringe is used it may be filled with carbon dioxid or oxygen gas according to the preference or facilities of the operator. When the syringe or bulb is used in connection with a manometer there is additional evidence of patency or nonpatency by the rise and fall of the pressure reading. When no pressure gage is used this evidence is lacking. In my original paper and in later publications I stated that in order to prove patency of the tubes there must be evidence in three directions: first, there must be a drop of pressure within certain limits during the insufflation; second, the patient must complain of shoulder symptoms; third, there must be proof of the presence of gas in the peritoneal cavity and most conveniently this may be seen under the diaphragm as a subphrenic pneumoperitoneum. When any one of these is absent one cannot be absolutely certain of the patency of the tubes.

1. If pressure alone is depended upon there may be a very fine leak along the cervical canal which might be inaudible to the examiner. There may be a fine leak in the apparatus itself, in the tubing or the attachments, and if not enough gas is introduced there will be absence of shoulder symptoms which in these simplified methods are commonly depended upon to demonstrate the fact of patency of the fallopian tubes.

2. The matter of the quantity of gas to be insufflated is of great importance especially when the small bulb or small syringe is used. It has been demonstrated repeatedly that at least 10 to 15 c.c. of gas under pressure is required to pass through the tubes. With the possibilities of leakage, back along the cervical canal, this small quantity of air can frequently lead to error. Even where the manometer shows a decline in pressure at a certain point this decline may be accounted for by a leak at the point of attachment between cannula and bulb or along the cervical canal or at any of the attachments in the apparatus. As long as the gas is not under appreciable pressure a minute defect in the apparatus may be responsible for the negligible amount of leakage. As soon as the pressure is raised to a point sufficient to overcome uterine and tube resistance the gas escapes through the tiniest defect. This is very well illustrated in the difference between allowing air or gas under the same pressure-flow ratio to pass into a collapsible, easily distensible rubber balloon with a capacity, let us say, of 500 c.c. and a thick, less distensible, and more resistant hollow muscular organ with a much smaller capacity, as the uterus. The latter will take 10 to 15 or 20 c.c. registering pressures varying from 20 to 200 mm. Hg, while this same amount in the balloon would up to that point practically register atmospheric pressure. The collapsible balloon may contain 10 or 15 c.c. of air though there be a small rent in some part of it. Again it must be remembered that the uterus reacts against the inflow of gas by contracting. This it does in the presence of patent or nonpatent tubes. When the tubes are open the gas flows into the peritoneal cavity and no more than 20 to 30 mm. Hg is required to keep up the flow through the open fallopian tubes. When there is no yielding point of escape for the gas the pressure will continue to be high as long as the flow remains constant.

3. *Concerning shoulder symptoms;* pains in the shoulders after insufflation are pathognomonic. Yet there are a certain number of women, neuropathic in type who, in order to be accommodating, would reply affirmatively to the question as to whether they had pains in their shoulders. It is therefore absolutely necessary to check up this symptom by seeing the gas underneath the diaphragm by fluoroscopy. A roentgenograph may be insisted upon in doubtful cases when one or other of the factors involved in this diagnostic procedure has not been absolutely definite and clear.

4. Fluoroscopy may fail to show a small amount of gas while the x-ray plate can clearly demonstrate a slight subphrenic pneumoperitoneum.

All these points require but a few minutes to ascertain and when all are present one has precise knowledge of the fact of tubal patency or tubal occlusion. It must follow therefore that all so-called simplified methods which do not produce a subphrenic pneumoperitoneum and which do not occasion shoulder pains and have no provision for manometric control of pressure cannot be said to fulfill the requirements of the test and are therefore unreliable. It goes without saying, of course, that in some women the simplest procedure will be satisfactory. For example, whether the syringe or bulb is used a sufficient amount of gas is insufflated to occasion shoulder pains without requiring confirmation by the fluoroscope and without the manometer. The ideal patient for the simplified transuterine insufflation is one who is not inclined to be nervous and particularly a thin individual. In such a patient a very small amount of gas or air will cause both subphrenic pneumoperitoneum and also shoulder pains. In more obese patients a greater quantity of gas is required to cause these symptoms, and this factor has been taken into account almost from the beginning of my work. The amount of gas insufflated is proportional to the weight, height, and waistline of each patient. Finally when one takes into consideration the great variability and uncertainty of the nervous sensibilities and psychic reactions of the average patient it becomes clear that in transuterine insufflation as in other clinical diagnostic methods one had best depend largely upon the objective, physical evidence in each case.

When we come to consider the refinements in diagnosis such as, for example, normal patency, moderate stenosis, unilateral or bilateral occlusion or stenosis, it is absolutely necessary to have uniform, continuous flow of gas under a steady pressure rate. This fact is not generally appreciated by those to whom the practicability of this diagnostic test has appealed so far, and I would like again to emphasize the diagnostic value and importance of using a gas under a constant rate of flow and controlled by a manometer. The siphon meter which I first recommended in 1921 (Fig. 43) fulfills the requirement of volume measurement. It is automatic, accurate, and requires no handling once it is set up. The gas supply is provided by a small tank filled with carbon dioxid gas. The valve in this tank is so graduated as to deliver a constant even flow of gas at any speed required.

Experience with the specimen of the extirpated uterus has shown that in the normal uterus and tubes at least 40 mm. Hg are required before the gas passes from the uterine cavity through the uterine ostiæ of the tubes and out at the fimbria. In many cases this initial pressure rise is from 60 to 80 or even 100 mm. Hg. The speed with which this initial rise of pressure is registered depends upon the rapidity of flow of the gas. In other words, the faster the gas is introduced into the uterine cavity the faster will the initial pressure rise be reached. If this rate of gas is uniform, the same initial pressure rise will be noted every time an attempt is made in the same specimen to introduce gas through the tubes. Furthermore clinical experience has shown that when the gas is allowed to enter the uterine cavity at a rate of 15 seconds to raise the mercury column to 100 mm. Hg there is a certain degree of uniformity for the passage of the gas into and through the tubes. This rate-flow also occasions the slightest discomfort to the patient and gives uniform figures for comparison not only in many different patients, but also in the same patient when repeated on several occasions in case patency is not established at the first test.

Another way of regulating the pressure is to make the rate of water displacement in the siphon meter the chief criterion for the gas transmission. Thus, for example, it has been found that when 100 c.c. of gas is allowed to flow through the siphon meter in one minute, the time-pressure-rate flow ratio is almost the same as when the rise of pressure requires 15 seconds or 20 seconds time to reach 100 mm. Hg. The physical values are not exactly identical but practically and for clinical purposes they express the same thing. The chief significance of this criterion is the emphasis it lays upon *a slow and careful introduction of the gas* rather than an irregular uncertain and haphazard insufflation.

When under these conditions the initial rise recorded exceeds 100 mm. Hg, for example 120 to 160, and the gas nevertheless passes through into the peritoneal cavity, it must demonstrate the fact of some surmountable obstruction within the tube lumen, in other words a relative stricture. When on the other hand there is no uniform pressure-rate flow used and the other methods with *simpler* devices are depended upon, this high pressure may indicate normal patency or it may indicate anything at all. It will be borne in mind that no hand can produce a uniform pressure no matter how skilled. It is impossible to equal by hand pressure the inherent steadiness of pressure regulated by a mechanical device such as a fine valve. The significance of this fact was early appreciated in my work when I sought to simplify the apparatus and therefore resort was had to the siphon meter described in 1921. If one uses a syringe with a capacity of 150 c.c. one can introduce gas or air into the peritoneal cavity for all purposes, but it is not possible by this means to get the dependable uniform pressure rise which is obtainable by means of the gas tank. With the bulb this is even less possible.

In this connection it may also be stated that given these reliable factors it is possible to determine whether or not both tubes are freely patent and whether one tube or both are stenosed. In the normally patent tubes there is no complaint of lateral pain. When the patient complains of unilateral or bilateral pain it may be taken to indicate pressure distention of a portion of the tube proximal to the point of obstruction on one or both sides. This clinical observation has been of aid in answering the ever recurring question as to which tube is closed or stenosed, and has obviated the necessity of introducing opaque substances to determine the same thing. It is impossible without using a uniform pressure-rate flow of gas to determine these facts.

Another point of equal importance is the matter of safety secured by careful attention to the rate flow. Three accidents have been reported to me, one of which was unforeseen but avoidable; and the other two were both due to ignorance in the use of the method of transuterine insufflation. In the first instance a spectator brushed by the lever of the tank and released a great volume of gas under a terrific amount of pressure. The cannula being in place within the uterus, the tubes were seen to rupture near the fimbriated end.. Fortunately the patient was on the operating table, the abdomen being open. No harm resulted.

In another case the examiner allowed the gas to flow at a very fast rate and caused collapse by a terrific impact against the diaphragm of a large amount of gas rapidly delivered through the fallopian tubes. Bystanders watching this performance reported that the mercury within the manometer shot well up to the ceiling. It so happened that the patient selected for the test was a woman para-IV suffering from myocarditis and diabetes. The physician was a novice in the use of the method and had no clear idea of the procedure.

The third case was even less felicitous. This was a patient upon whom an amputation of the cervix had been performed some years before. The uterus contained several fibroid tumors, one, the largest, being the size of a large apple. The tubes had been converted into large hydrosalpinges. The physician not experienced with the test first dilated forcibly the cervical canal, insufflated the uterus with gas and then curetted. This is the order of the operation as stated by the physician in question. The patient became cyanotic and her respirations became embarrassed, anesthesia was not discontinued but the operator "quickly finished" the curettage. She ceased to breathe under the anesthetic and was not resuscitated. At the autopsy air was found in the pelvic veins, including those of the broad ligament, the inferior vena cava and the heart cavity. The tubes were found to be surrounded by adhesions widely distended and occluded at the fimbriated ends. The one tube was distended with blood and air. Without making further comment upon the operator it is clear that he was lacking not only in knowledge of the indications, contraindications, and technic of transuterine insufflation but also in gynecological pathology. It is difficult to imagine what he could have expected to accomplish by the curettage in the presence of non-patent tubes, which fact he must have ascertained if the test meant anything at all to him. It is not conceivable that the test was done correctly and interpreted as indicating patent tubes in the presence of the disease actually present. Moreover, had the insufflation been done by a competent man anesthesia would not have been necessary. Without this, the patient might have complained of faintness and the careful clinician would have desisted after a first unsuccessful attempt to force the gas through the closed tubes. On further inquiry into this case it developed that the operator had never performed transuterine insufflation before but had depended upon an interne to "shoot" the gas. Four attempts were thus made using high pressure each time.

In the original presentation of the test and subsequently it was emphasized that insufflation is not to be done in the presence of pelvic masses.

In this particular unfortunate case it may not be amiss to conjecture that the injury to the cervix occasioned by forcible dilatation of a stenosed cervical canal may have presented the avenue of entrance into the cervical veins and thence into the broad ligament, etc. Some of the gas held under pressure within the uterine cavity may have entered the general circulation after the endometrium was curetted, a fact demonstrated by Sampson with his bismuth experiments and in my own work. Too much stress cannot be laid upon this point of the necessity of slow, careful gas insufflation. It is striking that in the hands of the men who have employed transuterine insufflation according to all the rules of technic and indications, no such accident has occurred nor anything approaching a calamity and the number of insufflations may now be reckoned in the thousands. The two accidents just described have occurred in the hands of not only inexperienced but unqualified operators.

It has been urged particularly by continental authors that by using a small syringe, say 20 c.c. capacity, air embolism can be avoided because the uterine cavity permits of distention with 10 c.c. so that at most 5 or 10 c.c. would get into the veins. I have demonstrated that as much as 300 c.c. of gas can be introduced into the venous system without causing any harm provided, of course, the rate of injection is slow similar to that prescribed for transuterine insufflation. Nor does the amount of gas introduced via the uterus entail any essential danger within the peritoneum provided also that the rate of gas flow is slow and not in excess of 100 c.c. displacement per minute or faster than it requires to raise the mercury column to 100 mm. Hg within 15 or 20 seconds' time. On a number of occasions a large sized pneumoperitoneum has been produced by the transuterine route, injecting a liter or more. This has not been recommended as a routine measure by me since the primary interest in insufflation has been in its specific diagnostic value as a test of tubal patency; and for this only a diminutive pneumoperitoneum is necessary and adequate. It is a question of proper judgment in selecting the cases and of competent skill in using the technic no matter how simple this actually happens to be. As with everything else in medicine one should have precise knowledge of physiology and pathology in addition to a clear understanding of the object of any method in question. Simple as transuterine insufflation is and safe as it has proven in careful hands it may nevertheless lead to disaster when misemployed by careless and unskilled hands. It certainly is not recommended as a procedure to the average practitioner who has not been trained in gynecological procedures.

The bulb insufflation or the syringe insufflation without a manometer cannot be subscribed to because of its unreliability, nor can either of these methods with the addition of a manometer compare favorably with the volumanometer and uniform rate-flow auxiliary. The so-called simplified methods have perforce had the effect of lessening the degree of care to be exercised in the tubal patency test—a lack of care which cannot so readily attend the original method because one at least pays attention to the description of the technic and rules to be followed. But no matter what method is employed scrupulous regard must be had for the indications and contraindications, for the facts in physiology and pathology and with respect to the primary essentials of the technic itself, namely, slow and gentle gas flow avoiding trauma of any kind. *Trauma is so unessential* that the test is best carried out without any anesthesia; so little pain does it cause that the patient may have the test done in the physician's office. *This means, of course, that the case must be properly adapted for the test. There must be no bleeding present, no fever, no pelvic tenderness, tumors or purulent discharge. The patient must have no remote serious cardiac or respiratory disease.* It is obvious that aside from the possible dangers to such a debilitated patient there can be no good reason for prosecuting the test. These women are bad risks for pregnancy in any event and it is a rather idle pastime to subject them to transuterine insufflation. Yet in selected cases a diminutive subphrenic pneumoperitoneum even under these conditions can do no harm.

In case of doubt, it is well to take the patient's temperature before a thorough examination is made and to note the temperature at intervals for twenty-four hours after the examination. Experience with pelvic inflammatory disease has taught that in the presence of a subacute process, manipulation as by digital examination can evoke a rise of temperature. The same has been noted repeatedly in instances of conservative treatment where a patient leaves her bed too soon after an abatement of fever thus indicating inflammatory activity. The occurrence of menses with its attending hyperemia is a common cause of temperature rise in the course of adnexal disease. Other traumata of moderate or slight degree have been known to produce the same thing. In the interest of absolute safety therefore this added precaution may be taken and recourse may be had to the sedimentation test which has proved of aid in pointing to latent or subacute inflammmation.

In conclusion, the importance of gentleness in performing the test cannot be too emphatically stressed. The introduction of the cannula must occasion a minimum or negligible amount of pain or discomfort; it must follow the natural direction of the cervico-uterine curve as previously determined with sound and careful bimanual examination and must occasion no bleeding. When bleeding attends the insertion of the cannula, no further attempt should be made to go on with the test as it indicates an inflammatory condition of the endocervix and endometrium. This, to be sure, is a very rare occurrence, but it is better to defer the test for a more favorable time.

The time of preference has so far seemed to be from four to seven days after the complete cessation of the menstrual period. The endometrium is then in the resting stage and is least liable to infection though the latter is extremely remote in careful hands. By choosing the postmenstrual interval for uterine insufflation it will be possible always to avoid interfering with an existing uterine or extra-uterine pregnancy. This rule is of special value in cases of amenorrhea of shorter or longer duration where it is otherwise impossible, if the patient present herself several weeks after the last menstruation, to determine the length of gestation. As ovulation occurs not sooner than twelve to fourteen days from the onset of the last preceding menstruation, pregnancy cannot take place before this time and insufflation is theoretically and practically safest when done within a week after cessation of a regular menstruation. The theoretical possibility of endometrial dislocation as well as of embolism formation is also thus eliminated. Clinical and experimental observations have pointed to the advisability in any event of not exceeding a pressure of 200 to 250 mm. Hg. Higher pressures have been employed by experienced hands in the attempt to open tubes that had been previously demonstrated to be stenosed or closed. *It will not do for the beginner in this work,* and goes without saying that *such attempts are best undertaken under the most favorable auspices.* Finally by selecting the fourth to the seventh day the therapeutic possibilities of the test become increased while more uniform results as regards the pressure-rate-flow on the one side and tubal patency, stenosis, or occlusion on the other will be obtained.

In lieu of index the reader is referred to the voluminous Table of Contents in the first part of this volume.

(1)

www.ingramcontent.com/pod-product-compliance
Lightning Source LLC
LaVergne TN
LVHW011757200926
848484LV00003B/729